ABC OF DERMATOLOGY
EXPANDED TO INCLUDE EXTRA CHAPTERS
ON HOT CLIMATES

ABC OF DERMATOLOGY

INCLUDES EXTRA CHAPTERS

PAUL K BUXTON

Consultant Dermatologist
Royal Infirmary, Edinburgh, and Queen Margaret Hospital, Dunfermline

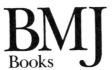

Books

In association with the Australian Medical Association

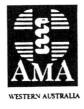

WESTERN AUSTRALIA

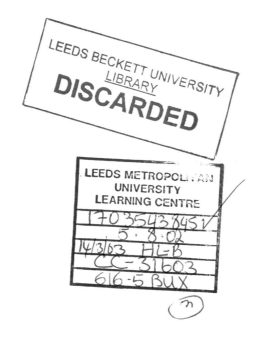
First published by the BMJ Publishing Group in 1988
Second impression 1989
Third impression 1990
Fourth impression 1991
Fifth impression 1991
Second edition 1993
Second impression 1994
Third impression 1994
Fourth impression 1996
Third edition 1998
Hot Climates edition 1999
Second impression June 1999
Third impression 2001
Fourth impression 2002
BMJ Publishing Group, BMA House, Tavistock Square,
London WC1H 9JR

British Library Cataloguing in Publication Data

A catalogue record for this book is avaialble from the British Library

ISBN 0-7279-1404-9

Cover illustration by Michael Courtney

Typeset by Apek Typesetters, Nailsea, Bristol
Printed and bound by Craft Print International Ltd, Singapore

CONTENTS

ACKNOWLEDGMENTS

Many colleagues have made useful comments on the original ABC of Dermatology articles and, where appropriate, changes have accordingly been made to the text. In some cases, however, the points raised related to specialised or controversial aspects which could not be discussed at length within the limits of an ABC.

This edition incorporates two new chapters by Professor R StC Barnetson, Professor of Dermatology, University of Sydney, Australia (UV Radiation and the Skin and Tropical Skin Diseases) and material contributed to the earlier editions by Dr DJ Gawkrodger, MD, FRCP, Consultant Dermatologist, Royal Hallamshire Hospital, Sheffield (Auto-immunity), DWS Harris, MRCP, Consultant Dermatologist, Whittington Hospital NHS Trust, London (Practical Procedures), D Kemmett, MRCP, Consultant Dermatologist, Vale of Leven Hospital, Dumbartonshire (Diseases of the Hair and Scalp), and Dr AL Wright, MRCP, Consultant Dermatologist, Bradford Royal Infirmary (Diseases of the Nails).

I am grateful to Dr Peter Ball, consultant in infectious diseases, for comments on infectious diseases, Dr M Jones, consultant in infectious diseases, for comments on parvovirus infections, and Mr C V Ruckley, consultantg surgeon, for comments on varicose ulcers.

The illustrations are from various sources including the Victoria Hospital, Kirkaldy, Queen Margaret Hospital, Dunfermline, and the Royal Infirmary, Edinburgh. A few were taken by the author.

The following colleagues kindly provided illustrations of specific conditions: Dr J A Savin, flea-bites on the ankle; Dr Peter Ball, rubella; Dr D H H Robertson, genital herpes; Mr C V Ruckley, varicose veins; Dr G B Colver, spider naevus; Dr M A Waugh and Dr M Jones, patients with AIDS; Dr P W M Copeman, common infections in black people; and Miss Julie Close, the diagrams of the nail and types of immune response.

Particular thanks are due to Mrs Mary Henderson for her patient and efficient typing and re-typing of the revisions for the text of this edition.

P K B

PREFACE

The skin is the major barrier between man and his environment and, being a dynamic relationship, more or less strain is placed on the skin as a result of changes in that relationship. Failure of that interface organ, i.e. the skin, is likely to lead to not only dermatological disease but also diseases of internal organs. In Australia, approximately one patient in ten who consults a general practitioner will do so for a skin disorder. In hot climates, with the increase in ambient temperature and, frequently, humidity, the skin tends to break down even more readily, with a consequent increase in the incidence of dermatological disease. As a result of increased awareness on the part of government and the public, as well as improved nutrition, better diagnostic methods, effective chemotherapy, and the full range of public health measures, certain diseases which were formerly common in more temperate areas have become increasingly restricted to hot climates. An example of this is leprosy which, at the turn of the century, was common in western Norway where Armaner Hansen, working in Bergen discovered the causal bacillus and gave his name to the disease. It is particularly fortunate that the author of the section on tropical skin diseases is Professor Ross Barnetson, Professor of Dermatology at the University of Sydney, who has conducted research into leprosy in Ethiopia and has also had practical experience of the management of tropical skin diseases as a medical officer in the British Army serving in Singapore.

Dermatolgoists working amongst Caucasian peoples in hot climates spend much of their time treating diseases caused by exposure to the sun. This includes the management of pre-malignant and malignant skin disease, both melanoma and non-melanoma skin cancer. They also treat many photosensitive disorders, such as photosensitive drug eruptions, and other forms of photosensitivity associated with internal disease. Other skin diseases that occur in both hot climates and more temperate ones, however, continue to make up the bulk of dermatological diseases seen in clinical practice. These include the eczema/dermatitis group of diseases, acne, psoriasis and the psoriasiform disorders, as well as various infections, including bacterial, viral and fungal. In recent years, the increasing knowledge of the mechanisms of dermatological disease has been aided, to a marked degree, by the great advances made in the basic sciences, particularly immunology.

Finally, there is little point in having knowledge without the ability to apply that knowledge in the treatment of patients. This work outlines a simple and effective approach to the patient with skin diseases and also basis instruction in some commonly used practical procedures.

William A Land
President of the Australasian College of Dermatologists

1. INTRODUCTION

The object of this book is to provide the dermatologist with a practical guide to the diagnosis and treatment of skin conditions. The symptoms, clinical appearance, and pathology of a few key common conditions are discussed. These are then used as a model for comparison with other skin diseases.

This approach is suitable for skin conditions that present with characteristic lesions such as blisters, ulceration, papules, or a rash. In other disorders, there may be a single causative factor that produces a variety of lesions, and it is more helpful to describe the characteristic clinical pattern that results. For example a drug reaction or auto-immune disease may produce widespread changes. Tumours, acne, leg ulcers, hair, and nails are covered as separate subjects.

The same condition is sometimes dealt with in more than one section, e.g. fungal infections are discussed under "Rashes with epidermal changes" and again under "Fungal and yeast infections". This repetition of the same topic from different perspectives should help in understanding it.

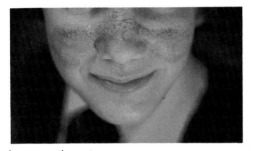

Lupus erythematosus.

One advantage of dealing with skin conditions is that the lesions are easily examined and can be interpreted without the need for complex investigations, although a biopsy is sometimes required to make or confirm the diagnosis. An understanding of the histological changes underlying the clinical presentation makes this interpretation easier and more interesting. Consequently, an account of the clinical appearances is correlated with underlying pathological changes.

Skin lesions are sometimes an indication of internal disease and may be the first clinical sign. For example, the girl in the photograph presented with a rash on her face, made worse by sunlight. She then mentioned that she was aware of lassitude, weight loss, and vague musculoskeletal symptoms which, in conjunction with the appearance of the rash, suggested lupus erythematosus. This was confirmed by further investigations and appropriate treatment initiated. Other dermatological associations with systemic disease are discussed in the relevant sections.

The significance of skin disease

A very large proportion of the population suffers from skin diseases, which make up approximately 1% of all consultations in primary care in the UK. However, community studies show that over 20% of the population have a medically significant skin condition and less than 25% of these had consulted a doctor.

The skin is not only the largest organ of the body, it also forms a living biological barrier and is the aspect of ourselves we present to the world. It is therefore not surprising that there is great interest in "skin care" with the associated vast cosmetic industry. The impairment of the normal functions of the skin can lead to acute and chronic illness with considerably disability and need for hospital treatment. Cancer arising in the skin can be fatal. A wide range of internal diseases, covering many different specialties, produces physical signs in the skin and there is the psychological effect of skin changes themselves on the individuals' personality. It is therefore important to use what Dr Papworth called "wide angle lenses" in assessing the patient and their disease. So in addition to concentrating on the individual lesion, the overall health and demeanour of the patient is taken into account. This also means making sure that there are no other signs, such as involvement of the nails, mucous membranes or other parts of the skin.

Descriptive terms

Macule

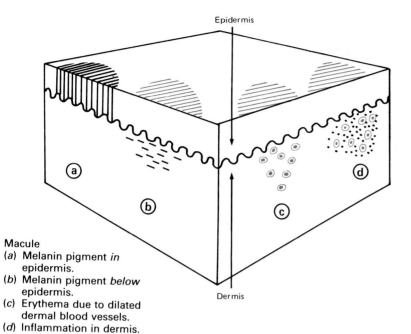

Macule
(a) Melanin pigment *in* epidermis.
(b) Melanin pigment *below* epidermis.
(c) Erythema due to dilated dermal blood vessels.
(d) Inflammation in dermis.

All specialties have their own common terms, and familiarity with a few of those used in dermatology is a great help. The most important are defined below.

Derived from the Latin for a stain, the term macule is used to describe changes in colour or consistency without any elevation above the surface of the surrounding skin. There may be an increase of melanin, giving a black or blue colour depending on the depth of the pigment. Loss of melanin leads to a white macule. Vascular dilatation and inflammation produce erythema (photograph below).

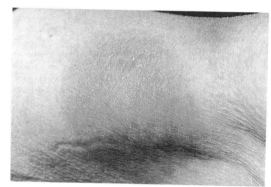

Papules and nodules

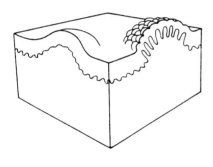

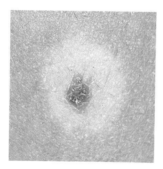

A papule surrounded by a depigmented macule.

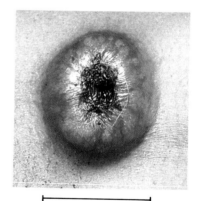

15mm

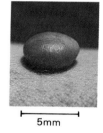

5mm

A papule is a circumscribed, raised lesion, conventionally less than 1 cm in diameter. It may be due to either epidermal or dermal changes.

A nodule is similar to a papule but over 1 cm in diameter.

Plaque

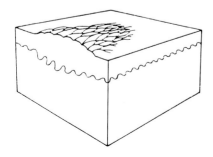

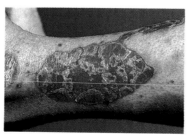

Plaque is one of those terms which convey a clear meaning to dermatologists but are often not understood by others. To take it literally, one can think of a commemorative plaque stuck on the wall of a building with a large area relative to its height and a well defined edge. Plaques are most commonly seen in psoriasis.

Vesicles and bullae

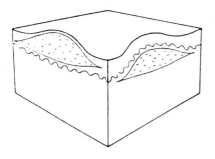 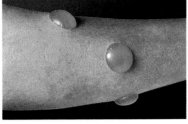

Vesicles and bullae are raised lesions that contain fluid. A bulla is a vesicle larger than 0·5 cm. They may be superficial within the epidermis or situated in the dermis below it.

Lichenification

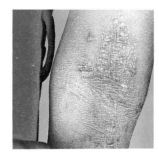

Lichenification is another term frequently used in dermatology as a relic of the days of purely descriptive medicine. Some resemblance to lichen seen on rocks and trees does occur, with hard thickening of the skin and accentuated skin markings. It is most often seen as a result of prolonged rubbing of the skin in localised areas of eczema.

Nummular lesions

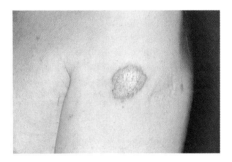

The word nummular literally means a "coin like" lesion. There is no hard and fast distinction from *discoid* lesions, which are flat disc like lesions of variable size. It is most often used to describe a type of eczematous lesion.

Pustules

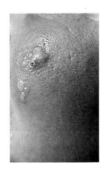

The term pustule is applied to lesions containing purulent material—which may be due to infection, as in the case shown, or sterile pustules are seen in pustular psoriasis.

Atrophy

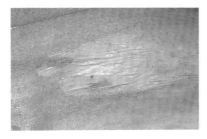

Loss of tissue may affect the epidermis, dermis, or subcutaneous fat. Thinning of the epidermis is characterised by loss of the normal skin markings, and there may be fine wrinkles, loss of pigment, and a translucent appearance. There may be other changes as well, such as sclerosis of the underlying connective tissue, telangiectasia, or evidence of diminished blood supply.

Introduction

Ulcer

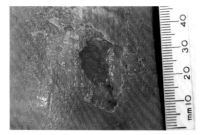

Ulceration results from the loss of the whole thickness of the epidermis and upper dermis. Healing results in a scar.

Erosion

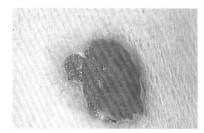

An erosion is a superficial loss of epidermis that generally heals without scarring.

Excoriation

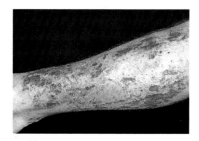

Excoriation is the partial or complete loss of epidermis as a result of scratching.

Fissuring

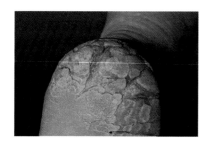

Fissures are slits through the whole thickness of the skin.

Annular lesions

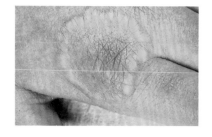

Annular lesions are ring shaped lesions.

Reticulate

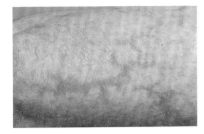

The term reticulate means "net like". It is most commonly seen when the pattern of subcutaneous blood vessels becomes visible.

Rashes

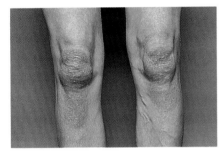

Psoriasis of both legs.

Approach to diagnosis

A skin rash generally poses more problems in diagnosis than a single, well defined skin lesion such as a wart or tumour. As in all branches of medicine a reasonable diagnosis is more likely to be reached by thinking firstly in terms of broad diagnostic categories rather than specific conditions.

If there is no history of a skin condition the rash is more likely to be due to an exogenous cause (such as contact dermatitis) than a constitutional condition (such as atopic eczema). Psoriasis can, however, appear in adults with no previous episodes. If several members of the household are affected a contagious condition should be considered (such as scabies). However, a common condition with a familial tendency, such as atopic dermatitis, may affect several family members at different times.

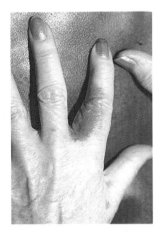

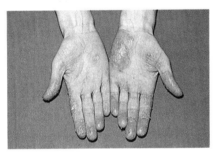

(Above) Symmetrical rash—irritant dermatitis.

(Left) Asymmetrical rash—contact dermatitis in a seamstress.

A simplistic but helpful approach to rashes is to clarify them as being from "inside" or "outside". Examples of "inside" or endogenous rashes are atopic eczema or drug rashes, whereas fungal infection or contact dermatitis are "outside" rashes. Although this distinction is not always clear cut, each type has distinctive characteristics.

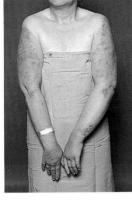

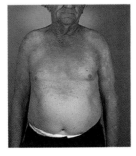

Allergic reactions producing photosensitivity. Note the areas protected by a vest in the patient on the right.

Symmetry

Most endogenous rashes affect both sides of the body, as in the atopic child or man with psoriasis on his knees. Of course, not all exogenous rashes are asymmetrical. A seamstress uses scissors in her right hand, where she may develop allergy to metal, but a hairdresser or nurse can develop contact dermatitis on both hands.

Distribution

It is useful to be aware of the usual sites of common skin conditions. These are shown in the appropriate sections. Eruptions that appear only on areas exposed to sun may, of course, be entirely or partially due to sunlight. Some conditions are due to a sensitivity to sunlight alone, such as polymorphous light eruption, or a photosensitivity to topically applied substances or drugs taken internally.

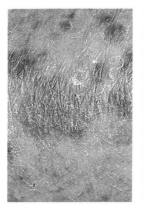

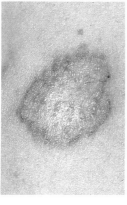

Lesion in deeper tissues with normal epidermis.

Small vesicles of eczema.

Morphology

The appearance of the skin lesion may give clues to the underlying pathological process.

The surface may consist of normal epidermis overlying a lesion in the deeper tissues. This is characteristic of many types of erythema in which there is dilatation of the dermal blood vessels associated with inflammation. The skin overlying cysts or tumours in the dermis and deeper tissues is usually normal. Conditions affecting the epidermis will produce several visible changes such as thickening of the keratin layer and scales in psoriasis or a more uniform thickening of the epidermis in areas lichenified by rubbing. An eczematous process is characterised by small vesicles in the epidermis with crusting or fine scaling.

The margin of some lesions is very well defined, as in psoriasis or lichen planus, but in eczema it merges into normal skin.

Blisters or vesicles occur as a result of (*a*) oedema between the epidermal cells or (*b*) destruction of epidermal cells or (*c*) the result of separation of the epidermis from the deeper tissues. Of course, more than one mechanism may occur in the same lesion. Oedema within the epidermis is seen in endogenous eczema, although it may not be apparent clinically, particularly if it is overshadowed by inflammation and scaling. It is also a feature of contact dermatitis. Widespread blisters occur in:

(*a*) viral diseases such as chickenpox; hand, foot, and mouth disease; and herpes simplex;

(*b*) bacterial infections such as impetigo;

(*c*) primary blistering disorders such as dermatitis herpetiformis, pemphigus, pemphigoid, metabolic disorders such as porphyria.

Bullae may occur in congenital conditions (such as epidermolysis bullosa), lichen planus, and pemphigoid without much inflammation. On the other hand, those forming as a result of vasculitis, sunburn, or an allergic reaction may be associated with pronounced inflammation. In pustular psoriasis there are deeper pustules, which contain polymorphs but are sterile and show little inflammation. Drug rashes can appear as a bullous eruption.

Induration is thickening of the skin due to infiltration of cells; granuloma formation; or deposits of mucin, fat, or amyloid.

Inflammation is indicated by erythema, which may be accompanied by increased temperature if acute—for example, in cellulitis or erythema nodosum. Chronic inflammatory cells may be present in conditions such as lichen planus or lupus erythematosus.

Eczema—intraepidermal vesicle

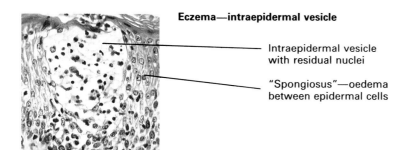

Intraepidermal vesicle with residual nuclei

"Spongiosus"—oedema between epidermal cells

Pemphigus—destruction of epidermal cells

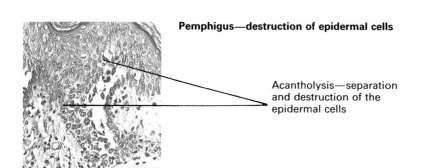

Acantholysis—separation and destruction of the epidermal cells

Pemphigoid—blister forming below epidermis

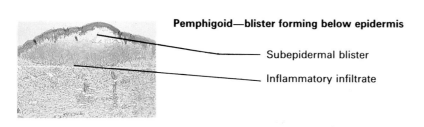

Subepidermal blister

Inflammatory infiltrate

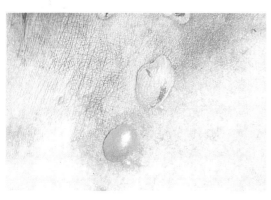

Pemphigus—superficial blister.

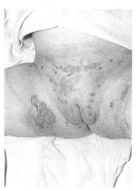

Herpes simplex.

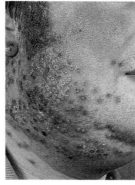

Impetigo.

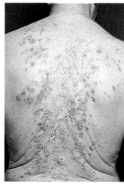

Dermatitis herpetiformis.

Assessment of the patient

A relevant history should be taken with particular reference to:

Where? Site of initial lesion(s) and subsequent distribution.

How long? Has the condition been continuous or intermittent?

Prognosis Is it getting better or worse?

Previous episodes How long ago? Were they similar? Have there been other skin conditions?

Who else? Are other members of the family affected? Or colleagues at work or school?

Other features Is there itching, burning, scaling, or blisters? Any associated factors, drugs, associated illnesses? Any effect of occupation, or home environment?

Treatment By prescription or over the counter?

Patients should be examined with particular reference to:

Distribution—This may give the essential clue, so a full examination is necessary. For example, there are many possible causes for dry thickened skin on the palms, and finding typical psoriasis on the elbows, knees, and soles may give the diagnosis.

Morphology—Are the lesions dermal or epidermal? Macular (flat) or forming papules? Indurated or forming plaques? With a well defined edge? Forming crusts, scabs, or vesicles?

Pattern—This is the overall clinical picture of both morphology and distribution. For example, an indeterminate rash may be revealed as pityriasis rosea when the "herald patch" is found.

We now come to the matter of using these basic concepts in the diagnosis of lesions in practice. In the next four chapters two common skin diseases are considered—psoriasis, which affects 1–2% of the population, and eczema, an even more common complaint. Both are rashes with distinctive epidermal changes. The difficulty arises with the unusual lesion: Is it a rarity or a variation of a common disease? What should make us consider further investigation? Is it safe to wait and see if it resolves or persists? The usual clinical presentations of psoriasis and eczema are also used as a basis for comparison with variations of the usual pattern and other skin conditions.

The effect of a skin condition on the patient's life and the patient's attitude to it must always be taken into account. For example, severe pustular psoriasis of the hands can be devastating for a self employed electrician and total hair loss from the scalp very distressing for a 16 year old girl.

Fear that a skin condition may be due to cancer or infection is often present and reassurance should always be given whether asked for or not. If there is the possibility of a serious underlying cause that requires further investigation it is part of good management to answer any questions the patient has and provide an explanation that he or she can understand. We all forget this aspect of medical practice at times.

The role of occupational factors must be remembered: dermatitis of the hands often means a hairdresser must change her job whereas it may be readily controlled in a teacher.

Patients understandably ask whether psoriasis can be cured and often want to know the cause. The cause is unknown and the best answer is that the tendency to develop psoriasis is part of a person's constitution and some factor triggers the development of the clinical lesions. Known factors include physical or emotional stress, local trauma to the skin (Koebner's phenomenon), infection (in guttate psoriasis), drugs (β blockers, lithium, and antimalarial drugs).

Further reading

Braun-Falco O, Plewig G, Wolff HH, Winkelmann RK. *Dermatology*. Berlin: Springer-Verlag, 1991.
Champion RH, Burton JL, Ebling FJ. *Textbook of dermatology*. 5th ed. Oxford: Blackwell Scientific, 1992.
Fitzpatrick TB, Freedberg IM, Eisen AZ, Austen KF, Wolff K. *Dermatology in general medicine*. 4th ed. New York: McGraw-Hill, 1993.
Sams WM, Lynch PJ, editors. *Principles and practice of dermatology*. 2nd ed. New York: Churchill Livingstone, 1996.

2. PSORIASIS

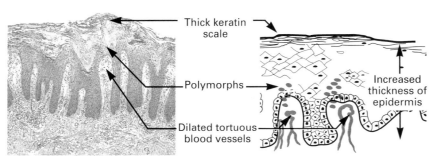

Increased epidermal proliferation—nuclei found . . . throughout the epidermis.

The familiar pink or red lesions with a scaling surface and well defined edge are easily recognised. These changes can be related to the histological appearance:

(1) The increased thickness of the epidermis, presence of nuclei above the basal layer, and thick keratin are related to increased epidermal turnover.

(2) Because the epidermis is dividing it does not differentiate adequately into normal keratin scales. These are readily removed to reveal the tortuous blood vessels beneath—clinically, "Auspitz sign". The psoriatic plaque can be likened to a brick wall badly built by a workman in too much of a hurry—it may be high but it is easily knocked down.

(3) The polymorphs that migrate into the epidermis form sterile pustules in pustular psoriasis. These are most commonly seen on the palms and soles.

(4) The dilated blood vessels can be a main feature, giving the clinical picture of intense erythema.

The equivalent changes in the nail cause thickening and "pits" 0·5–1·0 mm in diameter on the surface; these are thought to be due to small areas of psoriatic changes in the upper nail plate that then fall out. Onycholysis, in which the nail plate is raised up, also occurs in psoriasis.

While still considering the individual lesion remember the following points.

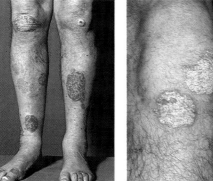

Plaques of psoriasis.

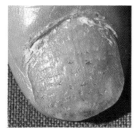

Pitting of nail.

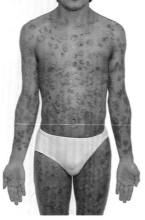

Small and large lesions.

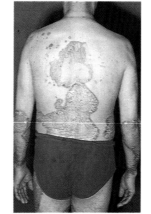

The *size* of the lesions varies from a few millimetres to very extensive plaques.

Scaling may predominate, giving a thick plaque, which is sometimes likened to limpets on the sea shore, hence the name "rupioid." Scratching the surface produces a waxy appearance—the "tache de bougie" (literally "a line of candle wax").

Erythema may be conspicuous, especially in lesions on the trunk and flexures.

Pustules are rare on the trunk and limbs, but deep seated pustules on the palms and soles are fairly common.

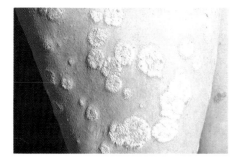

Rupioid lesions

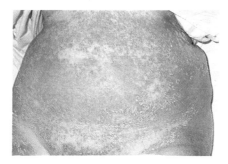

Widespread pustular psoriasis.

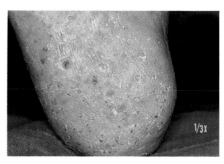

Pustules on the sole.

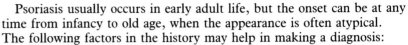

The typical patient

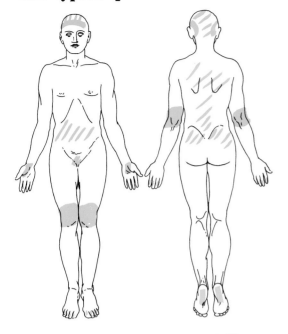

Psoriasis usually occurs in early adult life, but the onset can be at any time from infancy to old age, when the appearance is often atypical. The following factors in the history may help in making a diagnosis:

- There may be a family history—if one parent has psoriasis 16% of the children will have it, if both parents the figure is 50%
- The onset can occur after any type of stress, including infection, trauma, or childbirth
- The lesions may first appear at sites of minor trauma—Köebner's phenomenon
- The lesions usually clear on exposure to the sun
- Typically, psoriasis does not itch
- There may be associated arthropathy—affecting either the fingers and toes or a single large joint.

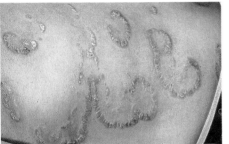

Annular lesions.

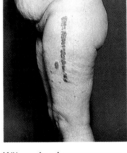

Köbner's phenomenon: psoriasis in surgical scar.

Clinical presentation

Patients usually present with plaques and sometimes annular lesions on the elbows, knees, and scalp. Patients with psoriasis show Köbner's phenomenon with lesions developing in areas of skin trauma such as scars or minor scratches. Normal everyday trauma such as handling heavy machinery may produce hyperkeratotic lesions on the palms. In the scalp there is scaling, sometimes producing very thick accretions. Erythema often extends beyond the hair margin. The nails show "pits" and also thickening with separation of the nail from the nail bed (oncholysis).

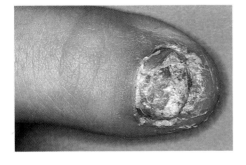

Psoriasis of the nail.

Variations

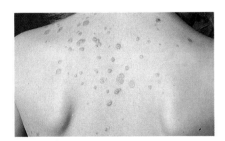

Guttate psoriasis.

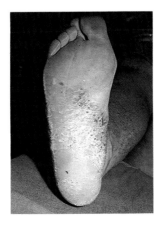

Pustules on the foot.

Guttate psoriasis—from the Latin *gutta*, a drop—consists of widespread small pink macules that look like drops of paint. It usually occurs in adolescents and often follows an acute β haemolytic streptococcal infection. There may be much distress to both parent and child when a previously healthy adolescent erupts in apparent leprous spots.

Pustular lesions occur as chronic deep seated lesions on the palms and soles with surrounding erythema which develop a brown colour and scaling. In clinics north of the border these pustules make the patient ask whether the condition is "smitten"—that is, infectious. It is important always to explain that it is not.

Psoriasis

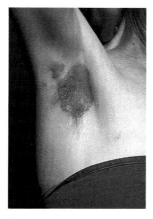

Flexural psoriasis.

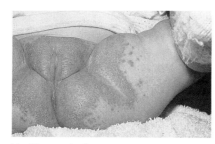

Napkin psoriasis.

Flexural psoriasis produces well defined erythematous areas in the axillae and groins and beneath the breasts. Scaling is minimal or absent.

Napkin psoriasis in children may present with typical psoriatic lesions or a more diffuse erythematous eruption with exudative rather than scaling lesions.

Generalised pustular psoriasis is uncommon. Superficial pustules develop in an area of intense erythema.

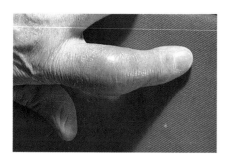

Erythrodermic psoriasis.

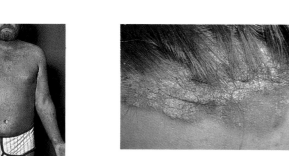

Scalp psoriasis.

Erythrodermic psoriasis is a serious, even life threatening, condition with erythema affecting nearly the whole of the skin. Diagnosis may not be easy as the characteristic scaling of psoriasis is absent, although this usually precedes the erythroderma. Less commonly the erythema develops suddenly without preceding lesions. There is a considerable increase in cutaneous blood flow, heat loss, metabolism, and water loss.

It is important to distinguish between the *stable*, chronic, plaque type of psoriasis, which is unlikely to develop exacerbations and responds to tar, dithranol, and ultraviolet treatment, and the more *acute* erythematous type, which is unstable and likely to spread rapidly, particularly when irritated by tar, dithranol, or ultraviolet light.

Joint disease in psoriasis

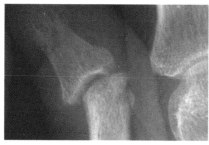

Acute arthropathy.

Patients with seronegative arthropathy of the non-rheumatoid type show double the normal (2%) incidence of psoriasis. Psoriatic arthropathy commonly affects the distal interphalangeal joints, sparing the metacarpophalangeal joints, and is usually asymmetrical. Rheumatoid nodules are absent. The sex ratio is equal but a few patients develop a "rheumatoid like" arthropathy, which is more common in women than in men. There is a third rare group who suffer from arthritic changes, in which there is considerable resorption of bone.

Other members of the families of those with psoriatic arthropathy are affected in 40% of cases.

There may be severe pustular psoriasis of the fingers and toes associated with arthropathy. One patient was so severely affected that she was immobilised until her condition cleared on treatment with methotrexate.

Causes of psoriasis

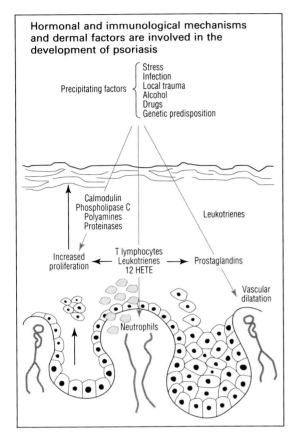

Hormonal and immunological mechanisms and dermal factors are involved in the development of psoriasis

Precipitating factors
- Stress
- Infection
- Local trauma
- Alcohol
- Drugs
- Genetic predisposition

Calmodulin
Phospholipase C
Polyamines
Proteinases

Leukotrienes

Increased proliferation

T lymphocytes
Leukotrienes
12 HETE

Prostaglandins

Vascular dilatation

Neutrophils

The cause is unknown but there is an inherited predisposition. Local trauma, acute illness, and stress may be factors in causing the appearance of clinical lesions. β haemolytic streptococcal throat infection is a common precipitating factor in guttate psoriasis. Antimalarial drugs, lithium, and β blockers can make psoriasis worse. There is evidence that psoriasis occurs more readily and is more intractable in patients with a high intake of alcohol. Smoking is associated with palmo-plantar pustulosis.

There is evidence that both hormonal and immunological mechanisms are involved at a cellular level. The raised concentrations of metabolites of arachodonic acid in the affected skin of people with psoriasis are related to the clinical changes. Prostaglandins cause erythema, while leukotrienes (LTB4 and 12 HETE) cause neutrophils to accumulate. The common precursor of these factors is phospholipase A2, which is influenced by calmodulin, a cellular receptor protein for calcium. Both phospholipase A2 and calmodulin concentrations are raised in psoriatic lesions.

T helper lymphocytes have been found in the dermis as well as antibodies to the basal cell nuclei of psoriatic skin. There are also dermal factors that contribute to the development of psoriatic lesions.

The detailed treatment of psoriasis is covered in the next chapter. The only point to be made here is the importance of encouraging a positive attitude with expectation of improvement but not a permanent cure, since psoriasis can recur at any time. Some patients are unconcerned about very extensive lesions while to others the most minor lesions are a catastrophe.

Further reading

Farber EM. *Psoriasis.* Amsterdam: Elsevier, 1987.
Fry L. *An atlas of psoriasis.* London: Parthenon Publications, 1992.
Mier PD, Van de Kerkhof PC. *Textbook of psoriasis.* Edinburgh: Churchill Livingstone, 1986.
Roenigk HH, Maibach HI. *Psoriasis.* Basle: Dekker, 1991.

3. TREATMENT OF PSORIASIS

It vanished quite slowly, beginning with the end of the tail, and ending with the grin, which remained some time after the rest of it had gone.

LEWIS CARROLL, *Alice in Wonderland*

Presentation of psoriasis	Treatment of choice	Alternative treatment
Stable plaque	Short contact dithranol	Tar
Extensive stable plaque	PUVA + etretinate	Short contact dithranol
Widespread small plaque	Ultraviolet B	Tar
Guttate psoriasis	Emollients while erupting then ultraviolet B	Weak tar preparations
Facial psoriasis	1% Hydrocortisone ointment	
Flexural psoriasis	Local mild to moderate strength steroids + antifungal	
Pustular psoriasis of hands and feet	Moderate to potent strength local steroid	Acitretin
Acute erythrodermic, unstable, or generalised pustular psoriasis	Inpatient treatment with ichthammol paste. Local steroids may be used in skilled hands	Methotrexate

To ignore the impact of the condition on the patient's life is to fail in treating psoriasis. Like the Cheshire cat that Alice met, it tends to clear slowly and the last remaining patches are often the hardest to clear.

This is frustrating enough but there is also the knowledge that it will probably recur and need further tedious courses of treatment. So encouragement and support are an essential part of treatment.

Treatment comprises local treatment with ointments and pastes, systemic drugs, or various forms of ultraviolet light. This should suit the type of psoriasis. The age and health of the patient, social and occupational factors need to be taken into consideration. The motivation of the individual patient is also important.

The preparations mentioned in the text are listed in the formulary at the end of the book.

It is estimated that 80% of patients with psoriasis do not consult a doctor, as the lesions are minimal.

Local treatment

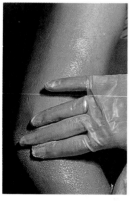
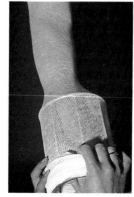
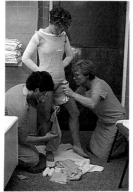
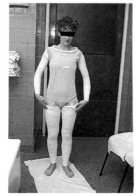

Local treatments entail the use of ointments and pastes, usually containing tar in various forms. It is much easier to apply them in hospital than at home if patients can make the time for hospital visits. Inpatient treatment can be more intensive and closely regulated; it also has the advantage of taking the patient completely away from the stresses of the everyday environment. In some units a "five day ward" enables patients to return home at weekends, which is particularly important for parents with young children.

Coal tar preparations are safe and effective for the stable plaque-type psoriasis but will irritate acute, inflamed areas. On the other hand, tar may not be strong enough for thicker hyperkeratotic lesions. Salicylic acid, which helps dissolve keratin, can be used in conjunction with tar for thick plaques. Refined coal tar extracts can be used for less severe areas of psoriasis.

Ichthammol, prepared from shale rather than coal tar, is less irritating and has a soothing effect on inflamed skin. It is therefore useful for "unstable" or inflamed psoriasis, when tar would not be tolerated.

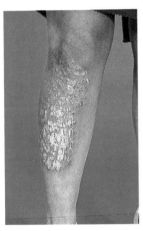

Psoriasis suitable for short contact dithranol treatment.

Dithranol, obtained originally from the Goa tree in south India, is now made synthetically. It can easily irritate or burn the skin, so it has to be used carefully and should be kept from contact with normal skin as far as possible. For hospital treatment pastes are used and the lesions surrounded by vaseline to protect the normal skin. Dithranol creams can be used at home—they are applied for 30 minutes and then washed off. A low concentration (0·1%) is used initially and gradually increased to 1% or 2% as necessary. All dithranol preparations are irritants and produce a purple-brown staining that clears in time. If used in the scalp it stains red or fair hair purple.

Emollients soften dry skin and relieve itching. They are a useful adjunct to tar or dithranol.

Corticosteroid preparations produce an initial clearing of psoriasis, but there is rapid relapse when they are withdrawn and tachyphylaxis (increasing amounts of the drug have a diminishing effect) occurs. Strong topical steroids should be avoided. Only weak preparations should be used on the face but moderately potent steroids can be used elsewhere: (*a*) if there are only a few small lesions of psoriasis; (*b*) if there is persistent chronic psoriasis of the palms, soles, and scalp (in conjunction with tar paste, which is applied on top of the steroid at night); and (*c*) in the treatment of psoriasis of the ears, flexures, and genital areas. In flexural psoriasis secondary infection can occur and steroid preparations combined with antibiotics and antifungal drugs should be used, such as Terra-Cortril with nystatin and Trimovate.

Calcipotriol and *Talcacitol*, vitamin D analogues, are calmodulin inhibitors used topically for mild or moderate plaque psoriasis. They are available as non-staining creams that are easy to use but can cause irritation. Sometimes a plateau effect is seen with the treatment becoming less effective after an initial response. In this case, other agents, such as tar preparations, have to be used as well to clear the lesions completely. It is important to observe the maximum recommended dose so as to prevent changes in calcium metabolism.

Ultraviolet treatment

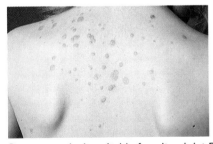

Guttate psoriasis suitable for ultraviolet B treatment.

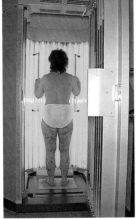

PUVA cabinet.

Ultraviolet B is short wavelength ultraviolet light and is used for widespread thin lesions or guttate psoriasis. The dose has to be accurately controlled to give enough radiation to clear the skin without burning. Recently, "narrow waveband" ultraviolet B treatment has been developed, which increases the therapeutic effect and diminishes burning. It can be used instead of PUVA in many cases.

Ultraviolet A is long wavelength ultraviolet light, which is effective if combined with systemic psoralens (PUVA): 8-methoxypsoralen (0·6–0·8 mg/kg body weight) is taken one to two hours before treatment.

After medical assessment treatment is given two or three times a week, with gradually increasing doses of ultraviolet A, given in a specially designed cabinet. Once the psoriasis has been cleared maintenance treatments can be continued once every two or three weeks. Protective goggles are worn during treatment with ultraviolet A and opaque glasses for 24 hours after each treatment.

Treatment of psoriasis

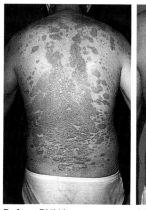 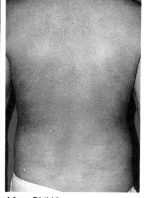

Before PUVA.   After PUVA.

A variable degree of erythema and itching may occur after treatment. Longer term side effects include a slight risk of epitheliomas developing, premature aging of the skin, and cataract formation (which can be prevented by wearing ultraviolet A filtering goggles during and after treatment). The total cumulative dosage is carefully monitored and kept as low as possible to reduce the risk of side effects.

Systemic treatment

Extensive and inflamed psoriasis that is resistant to local treatment may require systemic treatment. Although a number of antimetabolite drugs (such as azathioprine and hydroxyurea) and immunosuppressive drugs (such as cyclosporin A) are used, methotrexate and acitretin are the most useful.

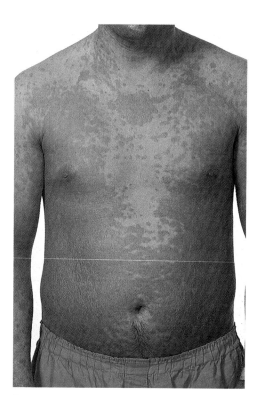

Erythematous psoriasis suitable for methotrexate treatment, having failed to respond to PUVA.

Methotrexate inhibits folic acid synthesis during the S phase of mitosis and diminishes epidermal turnover in the lesions of psoriasis. Because it is hepatotoxic liver function has to be assessed initially and at regular intervals during treatment. The dosage must be monitored and when a total of 1·5 g is reached a liver biopsy is indicated to exclude significant liver damage. An initial test dose is followed by a full blood count and if this gives normal results a weekly dose of 7·5–15 mg is used. As it is excreted in the urine the dose must be reduced if renal function is impaired. Aspirin and sulphonamides diminish plasma binding. It may interact with barbiturates, para-aminobenzoic acid, phenytoin, probenecid, phenylbutazone, oral contraceptives, and colchicine.

Acitretin is a vitamin A derivative that can be prescribed only in hospital in the United Kingdom. It is useful in pustular psoriasis and has some effect on other types of psoriasis. However, the effect is increased when combined with PUVA. Minor side effects include drying of the mucous membranes, crusting in the nose, itching, thinning of the hair, and erythema of the palms and nail folds. These are usually not severe and settle when treatment stops. More significant side effects include hepatotoxicity and raised lipid concentrations. Liver function tests and serum lipid (cholesterol and triglyceride) concentrations have to be carefully monitored. Etretinate is teratogenic and should not normally be used in women during reproductive years. If it is effective contraception must be used during treatment and for two years afterwards as the half life is 70–100 days.

Cyclosporin A is an immunosuppressant widely used following organ transplantation. It is effective in suppressing the inflammatory types of psoriasis. Blood tests should be carried out before starting treatment, particularly serum creatinine, urea, and electrolyte, as cyclosporin A can interfere with renal function.

Psoriasis of the scalp

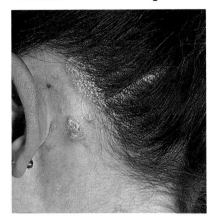

- Scalp psoriasis can be very difficult to clear, particularly if there are thick scales

- 3% Salicylic acid in a suitable base and left on for four to six hours or overnight and then washed out with a tar shampoo

- Dithranol preparations are effective but tint blonde or red hair purple

- Steroid preparations can be used to control itching

Further reading

Lowe NJ. *Managing your psoriasis*. London: Master Media, 1993.
Lowe NJ. *Practical psoriasis therapy*. 2nd ed. St Louis, Mosby, 1992.

4. ECZEMA AND DERMATITIS

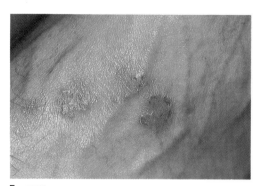

Eczema.

The terms eczema and dermatitis are interchangeable, covering a wide variety of conditions from the child with atopic eczema to the adult with an allergy to cement. "Eczema" is more specific and in some countries indicates a more acute condition than "dermatitis." If patients are told they have dermatitis they may assume that it is related to their employment with the implication that they may be eligible for compensation. It is not unusual for industrial workers to ask "Is it dermatitis doctor?"—meaning "is it due to my job?"

Clinical appearance

Eczema is an inflammatory condition of the skin characterised by groups of vesicular lesions with a variable degree of exudate and scaling. In some cases dryness and scaling predominate with little inflammation. In more acute cases there may be considerable inflammation and vesicle formation, in keeping with the Greek for "to boil out", from which the word eczema is derived. Sometimes the main feature may be blisters that become very large.

Eczema commonly itches and the clinical appearance may be modified by scratching, which with time may produce lichenification (thickening of the skin with increased skin markings). Also as a result of scratching the skin surface may be broken and have excoriations, exudate, and secondary infection.

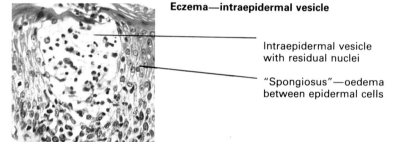

Eczema—intraepidermal vesicle

Intraepidermal vesicle
with residual nuclei

"Spongiosus"—oedema
between epidermal cells

Pathology

The characteristic change is oedema between the cells of the epidermis, known as spongiosus, leading to formation of vesicles. The whole epidermis becomes thickened with an increased keratin layer. A variable degree of vasodilatation in the dermis and an inflammatory infiltrate may be present.

Types of eczema

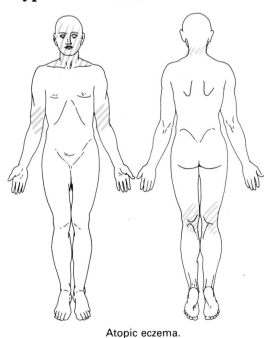

Atopic eczema.

The many causes of eczema are not consistently related to the distribution and clinical appearance. In general there are either external factors acting on the skin producing inflammatory changes or it is an endogenous condition. It is important to remember there can be more than one cause—for example, in atopic eczema or varicose eczema on the ankle an additional allergic reaction may develop to the treatments used.

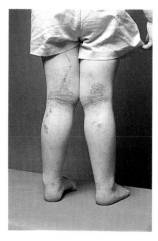

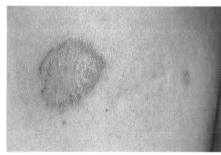

Nummular eczema.

Atopic eczema.

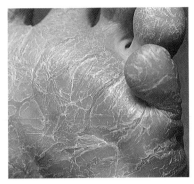

Plantar dermatosis.

Atopic eczema affects mainly the flexor surfaces of the elbows and knees and the face and neck. To a variable degree it can affect the trunk as well.

The typical patient with atopic eczema is a fretful scratching child with eczema that varies in severity, often from one hour to the next. In the older child or adult eczema is more chronic and widespread and its occurrence is often related to stress. Atopic eczema is common, affecting 3% of all infants, and runs a chronic course with variable remissions. It normally clears during childhood but may continue into adolescence and adult life as a chronic disease. It is often associated with asthma and rhinitis. Sufferers from atopic eczema often have a family history of the condition.

Variants of atopic eczema are pityriasis alba—white patches on the face of children with a fair complexion—and chronic juvenile plantar dermatosis—dry cracked skin of the forefoot in children. This does not affect the interdigital spaces and is not due to a fungal infection.

Eczema herpeticum—Children with atopic eczema are particularly prone to herpes virus infection, which may be life threatening. Close contact with adults with "cold sores" should therefore be avoided.

Nummular eczema appears as coin shaped lesions on legs and trunk.

Stasis eczema occurs around the ankles, where there is impaired venous return.

Paget's disease of the breast—While eczema of the nipples and areolae occur in women, any *unilateral*, persistent, areas of dermatitis in this region may be due to Paget's disease, in which there is underlying carcinoma of the ducts. In such cases a biopsy is essential.

Lichen simplex is a localised area of lichenification produced by rubbing.

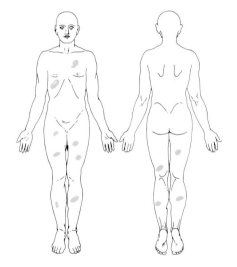

Nummular eczema.

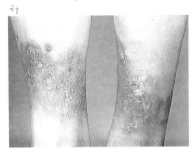

Stasis eczema.

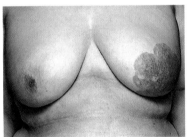

Paget's disease of the nipple.

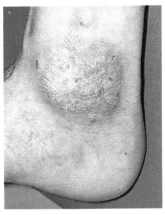

Lichen simplex.

Neurodermatitis is a term often used synonymously with lichen simplex. It is also used to describe generalised dryness and itching of the skin, usually in those with atopic eczema.

Asteatotic eczema occurs in older people with a dry, "crazypaving" pattern, particularly on the legs.

Pompholyx is itching vesicles on the fingers, with lesions on the palms and soles in some patients.

Infection can modify the presentation of any type of eczema or contact dermatitis.

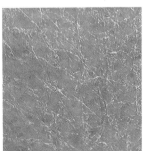

Asteatosis.

Pompholyx.

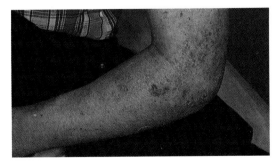

Infected eczema.

Contact dermatitis

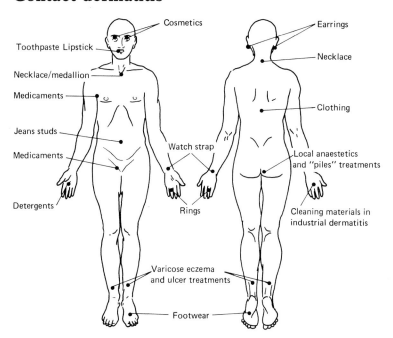

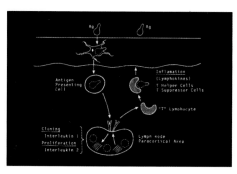

Common sources of allergic contact dermatitis

Jewellery, clothing, wristwatch, scissors, cooking utensils	Nickel—and cobalt occasionally
Cement, leather	Chromate
Hair dyes, tights, shoes	Paraphenylenediamine
Rubber gloves and boots	Rubber preservative chemicals
Creams, ointments, cosmetics	Preservatives (para-benz, quarternium), balsam of Peru, fragrances, lanolin neomycin, benzocaine, in medicated ointments

The skin normally performs its function as a barrier very effectively. If this is overcome by substances penetrating the epidermis an inflammatory response may occur leading to epidermal damage. These changes may be due to either (a) an allergic response to a specific substance acting as a sensitiser or (b) a simple irritant effect. An understanding of the difference between these reactions is helpful in the clinical assessment of contact dermatitis.

Allergic contact dermatitis

The characteristics of allergic dermatitis are:

- Previous exposure to the substance concerned.
- 48–96 hours between contact and the development of changes in the skin.
- Activation of previously sensitised sites by contact with the same allergen elsewhere on the body.
- Persistence of the allergy for many years.

The explanation of the sequence of events in a previously sensitised individual is as follows:

The antigen penetrates the epidermis and is picked up by a Langerhans cell sensitised to it. It is then transported to the regional lymph node where the paracortical region produces a clone of T cells specifically programmed to react to that antigen. The sensitised T cells accumulate at the site of the antigen and react with it to produce an inflammatory response. This takes 48 hours and is amplified by interleukins that provide a feedback stimulus to the production of futher sensitised T cells.

Allergic contact dermatitis can be illustrated by the example of an individual with an allergy to nickel who has previously reacted to a wrist watch. Working with metal objects that contain nickel leads to dermatitis on the hands and also a flare up at the site of previous contact with the watch. The skin clears on holiday but the dermatitis recurs two days after the person returns to work.

Irritant contact dermatitis

This has a much less defined clinical course and is caused by a wide variety of substances with no predictable time interval between contact and the appearance of the rash. Dermatitis occurs soon after exposure and the severity varies with the quantity, concentration, and length of exposure to the substance concerned. Previous contact is not required, unlike allergic dermatitis where previous sensitisation is necessary.

Photodermatitis, caused by the interaction of light and chemical absorbed by the skin, occurs in areas exposed to light. It may be due to (a) drugs taken internally, such as sulphonamides, phenothiazines, and dimethylchlortetracycline, or (b) substances in contact with the skin, such as topical antihistamines, local anaesthetics, cosmetics, and antibacterials.

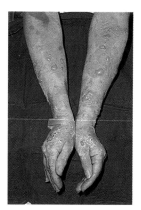

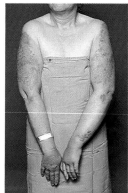

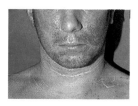

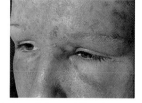

Allergic reactions to: (top left) sulphapyridine by mouth; (top right) Solarcaine and sun; (bottom left) topical neomycin; (bottom right) dithranol.

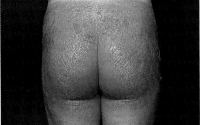

Acute irritant reaction to bleach.

Morphology—The clinical appearance of both allergic and irritant contact dermatitis may be similar but there are specific changes that help in differentiating them. An acute allergic reaction tends to produce erythema, oedema, and vesicles. The more chronic lesions are often lichenified. Irritant dermatitis may present as slight scaling and itching or extensive epidermal damage resembling a superficial burn, as the child in the illustration shows.

Pathology—The allergic reaction to specific sensitisers leads to a typical eczematous reaction with oedema separating the epidermal cells and blister formation. In irritant dermatitis there may also be eczematous changes but also non-specific inflammation, thickening of keratin, and pyknotic, dead epidermal cells.

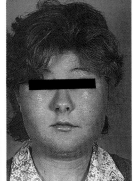

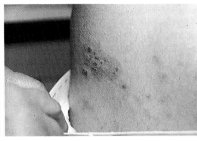

Allergic reactions to: (left) rubber pad on goggles; (middle) cosmetics; and (right) elastic in underpants.

The distribution of the skin changes is often helpful. For example, an itchy rash on the waist may be due to an allergy to rubber in the waistband of underclothing or a metal fastener. Gloves or the rubber lining of goggles can cause a persisting dermatitis. An irritant substance often produces a more diffuse eruption, as shown by the patient who developed itching and redness from dithranol.

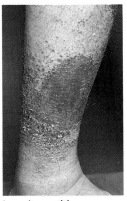

Leg dermatitis.

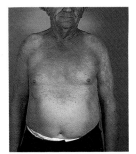

Photodermatitis.

Photodermatitis can occur from everyday household substances such as soap—the man in the photograph reacted to the trichlorsalicalanilide in soap he had used before working in his garden. The outline of the area protected by his vest can be seen.

Sensitisers in leg ulcer treatments

Neomycin
Lanolin (wool alcohol)
Formaldehyde
Tars
Chinaform (the "C" of many
  proprietary steroids)

An allergy to medications used for treating leg ulcers is a common cause of persisting dermatitis on the leg. Common allergens are listed in the box.

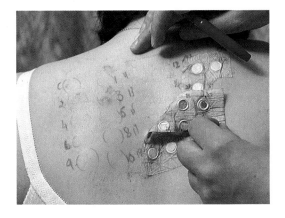

Patch testing

Patch testing is used to determine the substances causing contact dermatitis. The concentration used is critical. If it is too low there may be no reaction, giving a false negative result, and if it is too high it may produce an irritant reaction, which is interpreted as showing an allergy (false positive). Another possible danger is the induction of an allergy by the test substance. The optimum concentration and best vehicle have been found for most common allergens, which are the basis of the "battery" of tests used in most dermatology units.

The test patches are left in place for 48 hours then removed, the sites marked, and any positive reactions noted. A further examination is carried out at 96 hours to detect any further reactions.

Classification of eczema

Endogenous (constitutional) eczema

- Atopic
- Nummular/Discoid
- Pompholyx
- Stasis
- Seborrhoeic (discussed later)

Exogenous (contact) eczema

- Irritant
- Allergic
- Photodermatitis

Secondary changes

- Lichen simplex
- Neurodermatitis
- Asteatosis
- Pompholyx
- Infection

It is most important not to put a possible causative substance on the skin in a random manner without proper dilution and without control patches. The results will be meaningless and irritant reactions, which are unpleasant for the patient, may occur.

Further reading

Atherton DJ. *Eczema in childhood: the facts.* Oxford: Oxford University Press, 1994.
Cronin E. *Contact dermatitis.* Edinburgh: Churchill Livingstone, 1980.
Fisher AA. *Contact dermatitis.* 3rd ed. Baltimore: Williams & Wilkins, 1986.
Schwanitz HJ. *Atopic palmoplantar eczema.* Berlin: Springer-Verlag, 1988.

Occupational dermatitis

Dermatitis, which is simply inflammation of the skin, can arise as a result of:

Inherited tendency to eczema (atopy)
Contact dermatitis
  irritant
  allergic
Infection.

In the workplace, all three factors may be involved in causing dermatitis. For example, a student nurse or trainee hairdresser is exposed to water, detergents and other factors which will exacerbate any pre-existing eczema. In addition, there may be specific allergies and as a result of the broken skin, secondary infection can occur making the situation even worse. The following points are helpful in determining the role of occupational causes.

- If the dermatitis first occurred during employment or with a change of employment and had not been present before, then occupational factors are more likely.
- If the condition generally clears during holidays and when away from the workplace, this suggests an occupational cause, but chronic irritant dermatitis may persist when the patient is away from the workplace.
- If there is exposure to substances which are known to induce dermatitis and protective measures are inadequate.

If secondary infection is present, this can keep a dermatitis active even when away from the workplace and sometimes allergen exposure continues at home; for example, an allergy to rubber gloves at work will also occur when rubber gloves are used for domestic work at home.

Whatever the cause of the dermatitis, the end result may appear the same clinically, since the inflammation and blisters of atopic eczema may be indistinguishable from an allergic reaction to rubber gloves. Generally, contact dermatitis is more common on the dorsal surface of the hands while atopic eczema occurs on the palms and sides of the fingers.

Irritant contact dermatitis can occur acutely as mentioned above and there is usually a definite history of exposure to irritating chemicals.

Chronic irritant dermatitis can be harder to assess as it develops insidiously in many cases. Often it starts with episodes of transient inflammation that clear up, but with each successive episode the damage becomes worse with an escalation of inflammatory changes that eventually become chronic and fixed. This is shown graphically in the diagram in the margin.

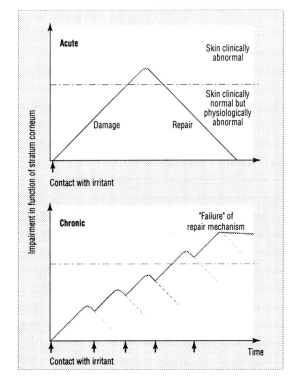

Once chronic damage has occurred the skin is vulnerable to any further irritation, so the condition may flare up in the future even after removal of the causative factors. Individuals with atopic eczema are particularly liable to develop chronic irritant dermatitis and secondary infection is an additional factor.

Allergic contact dermatitis occurs as an allergic reaction to specific substances. As this involves a cell mediated response the inflammatory reaction occurs about two days after exposure and once the allergy is present, further exposure will inevitably produce a reaction. Some substances are much more likely to produce an allergy, such as epoxy resin monomer, than others, such as cement, which characteristically carries exposure over many years before an allergy develops. In addition to the capacity of the substance to produce an allergic reaction, individuals also vary considerably in the capacity to develop allergies.

Immediate type sensitivity is sometimes seen as a reaction to food protein and sensitivity to latex gloves. This can produce a very severe reaction, particularly in atopic individuals.

Treatment of occupational dermatitis

The exact cause of the dermatitis should be identified as far as possible. It is important to ascertain exactly what an individual's job entails, e.g., a worker in a plastics factory had severe hand dermatitis but the only positive result on patch testing was to nickel. On visiting the factory it became clear that the cause was a nickel plated handle that he used several thousand times a day and not the plastic components that the machine was making. It is also important to assess the working environment, since exposure to damp and irritants (e.g., on an oil rig or in a coal mine) can irritate the skin.

If occupational factors are suspected, then a full assessment and investigation in a dermatology department is important as the patient's future working life may be at stake.

Further reading

Adams RM. *Occupational skin disease.* 2nd ed. Philadelphia: Saunders, 1990.
Arndt KA. *Manual of dermatological therapeutics.* 5th ed. New York: Little, 1995.
Foussereau J, Benezra JE, Maibach H. *Occupational contact dermatitis.* Copenhagen: Munksgaard, 1982.

> **Substances commonly causing allergic occupational dermatitis**
>
> - Chromate—in cement and leather
> - Biocides—e.g., formaldehyde and isothiazolinones, used in cutting oils in engineering
> - Epoxy resins—(uncured monomers)
> - Rubber chemicals
> - Hair dressing chemicals—particularly dyes and setting lotions
> - Plant allergens

The itching skin (pruritus)

It is sometimes very difficult to help a patient with a persistently itching skin, particularly if there is no apparent cause. Pruritus is a general term for itching skin, whatever the reason.

Itching with skin manifestations

Eczema is associated with itching due to the accumulation of fluid between the epidermal cells that are thought to produce stretching of the nerve fibres. As a result of persistent scratching there is often lichenification which conceals the original underlying areas with eczema. Exposure to irritants and persistent allergic reactions can produce intense itching and should always be considered.

"Allergic reactions" due to external agents often cause intense itching. Systemic allergic reactions such as a fixed drug eruption, erythema multiforme and vasculitis are less likely to cause pruritus.

Psoriasis, which characteristically has hyperkeratotic plaques, usually does not itch but sometimes there can be considerable itching. Occasionally this is due to secondary infection with breaks in the skin surface.

Lichen planus presents with groups of flat-topped papules which often cause an intense itch.

Blistering disorders of the skin may itch.

In *herpes simplex* there is usually burning and itching in the early stages.

In *herpes zoster* there may be a variable degree of itching but this is overshadowed by the pain and discomfort of the fully developed lesions. In contrast, bullous *impetigo* causes few symptoms, although there may be extensive blisters. Itching is usually not present.

Dermatitis herpetiformis is characterised by intense persistent and severe itching that patients often describe as being unendurable. Usual measures such as topical steroids and antihistamines have little if any effect. In contrast, the blisters of *pemphigoid* do not itch although the earlier inflamed lesions can be irritating.

Parasites—Fleas and mites cause pruritic papules in groups. The patient may not realise that they may have been acquired after a walk in the country or encountering

---

> **Systemic causes**
>
> *Endocrine diseases*—Diabetes, myxoedema, hyperthyroidism
> *Metabolic diseases*—Hepatic failure, chronic renal failure
> *Haematological*—Polycythaemia, iron deficiency anaemia
> *Malignancy*—Lymphoma, reticulosis, carcinomatosis
> *Psychological*—Anxiety, parasitophobia
> *Tropical infection*—Filariasis, hookworm
> *Drugs*—Alkaloids

Eczema and dermatitis

a dog or cat. *Nodular prurigo* may develop following insect bites and is characterised by persistent itching, lichenified papules, and nodules over the trunk and limbs. The patient attacks them vigorously and promotes a persisting "itch–scratch–itch" cycle which is very difficult to break.

Parasitophobia—This condition is characterised by the presence of small insects burrowing into the skin which persists despite all forms of treatment. The patient will produce small flakes of skin, fibres of clothing and pieces of dust usually in carefully folded pieces of paper for examination. These should always be examined and the patient gently informed that no insect could be found but this will not be believed. Treatment is therefore very difficult and sometimes recourse has to be had to psychotropic drugs such as pimozide which is a powerful drug and contraindicated in cardiac conditions.

Infestations with lice cause irritation and a scabies mite can cause widespread persistent pruritus, even though only a dozen or so active scabies burrows are present. It is always acquired by close human contact and the diagnosis may be missed unless an adequate history of personal contacts and a thorough clinical examination is carried out. On the other hand, a speculative diagnosis of scabies should be avoided.

Investigations

- Skin scrapings for mycology
- Patch testing for allergies
- Full blood count, erythrocyte sedimentation rate, liver and renal function tests
- Urine analysis
- Stools for blood and parasites

Itching with no skin lesions

If no dermatological lesions are present generalised pruritus or itchy skin may indicate an underlying internal cause. In the elderly, however, the skin may itch simply because it is dry.

Internal malignancy—Hodgkin's disease may present with pruritus long before any other manifestations. A 35-year-old ambulance driver attended the dermatology clinic with intense itching but a normal skin and no history of skin disease. His general health was good and both physical examination and all blood tests were normal. However, a chest X-ray film showed a mediastinal shadow that was found to be due to Hodgkin's lymphoma. Fortunately this was easily treated. Other forms of carcinoma rarely cause pruritus.

Metabolic and endocrine disease

Biliary obstruction and *chronic renal disease* cause intense pruritus. *Thyroid disease* can be associated with an itching skin. In hyperthyroidism the skin appears normal but in hypothyroidism there is dryness of the skin causing pruritus.

Blood diseases—Polycythaemia and iron deficiency are sometimes associated with itching skin.

Treatment

Treatment of the cause must be carried out when possible. Calamine lotion cools the skin with 0·5% menthol or 1% phenol in aqueous cream. Camphor-containing preparations and crotamiton (Eurax) are also helpful.

Topical steroid ointments and occlusive dressings may help to prevent scratching and may help to break the itch–scratch–itch cycle. Emollients should be used for dry skin.

Topical local anaesthetics may give relief but intolerance develops and they can cause allergic reactions. Sedative antihistamines at night may be helpful. In liver failure cholestyramine powder may help to relieve the intense pruritus, as this is thought to be due to bile salts in the skin.

Pruritus ani is a common troublesome condition and the following points may be helpful:

(1) Advise gentle cleaning once daily and patients should be advised to avoid excessive washing.

(2) Avoid harsh toilet paper, especially as it is coloured since cheap dyes irritate and cause allergies. Olive oil and cotton wool can be used instead.

(3) Weak topical steroids will help to reduce inflammation, with zinc cream or ointment as a protective layer on top.

(4) Anal leakage from an incompetent sphincter, skin tags, or haemorrhoids may require surgical treatment.

(5) There may be an anxiety or depression but prutitus ani itself can lead to irritability and depression.

Pruritus vulvae is a persistent irritation of the vulva which can be most distressing and is most common in post-menopausal women. It is important to eliminate any factors that may be preventing resolution, of which the most important are:

(1) Secondary infection with pyogenic bacteria or yeasts.

(2) Eczema or contact dermatitis.

(3) Lichen sclerosus atrophicus.

The adjacent vaginal mucosa should be examined to exclude an intraepithelial neoplasm or lichen planus.

Treatment includes suitable antiseptic preparations such as 2% eosin, regular but not excessive washing, emollients and topical steroids, bearing in mind the possibility of infection.

5. TREATMENT OF ECZEMA AND INFLAMMATORY DERMATOSES

(1) Treat the patient, not just the rash

(2) Avoid promising complete cure

(3) Be realistic about applying treatments at home

(4) Make sure the patient understands how to carry out the treatment

(5) Advise using emollients and minimal soap

(6) Provide detailed guidance on using steroids

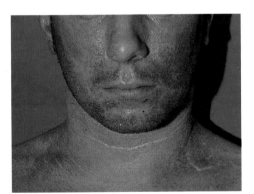

Weeping eczema.

Specific treatment

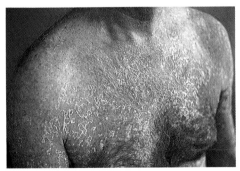

Acute erythema.

Treat the patient, not just the rash. Many patients accept their skin condition with equanimity but others suffer much distress—especially if the face and hands are affected. Acceptance by the doctor of the individual and his or her attitudes to the disease goes a long way to helping the patient live with the condition.

The common inflammatory skin diseases can nearly always be improved or cleared—but it is wise not to promise a permanent cure.

Be realistic about the treatment people can apply in their own homes. It is easy to unthinkingly give patients with a widespread rash a large amount of ointment to apply twice daily, which is hardly used because: (a) they have a busy job or young children and simply do not have time to apply ointment to the whole skin; (b) they have arthritic or other limitations of movement and can reach only a small part of the body; (c) the tar or other ointment is smelly or discolours their clothes. Most of us have been guilty of forgetting these factors at one time or another.

Dry skin tends to be itchy, so advise minimal use of soap. Emollients are used to soften the skin, and the simpler the better. Emulsifying ointment *BP* is cheap and effective but rather thick. I advise patients to mix two tablespoons in a kitchen blender with a pint of water—the result is a creamy mixture that can easily be used in the bath. A useful preparation is equal parts of white soft paraffin and liquid paraffin. Various proprietary bath oils are available and can be applied directly to wet skin. This is more sensible than putting them in the bath water, which makes the bath slippery with more oil going down the drain than on the skin. There are many proprietary emollients.

Steroid ointments are effective in relieving inflammation and itching but are not always used effectively. Advise patients to use a strong steroid (such as betamethasone or fluocinolone acetonide) frequently for a few days to bring the condition under control; then change to a weaker steroid (dilute betamethasone, fluocinolone, clobetasone, hydrocortisone) less frequently. Strong steroids should not be continued for long periods, and do not prescribe any steroid stronger than hydrocortisone for the face as a rule. Strong steroids can cause atrophy of the skin if used for long periods, particularly when applied under occlusive dressings. On the face they may lead to florid telangiectasia and acne like pustules. Avoid using steroids on ulcerated areas. Prolonged use of topical steroids may mask an underlying bacterial or fungal infection.

Wet, inflamed, exuding lesions

(1) Use wet soaks with normal saline or aluminium acetate (0·6%). Potassium permanganate (0·1%) solution should be used if there is any sign of infection.

(2) Use wet compresses rather than dry dressings.

(3) Steroid *creams* should be used as outlined above. Greasy ointment bases tend to float off on the exudate.

(4) A combined steroid-antibiotic cream is often needed as infection readily develops.

(5) Systemic antibiotics may be required in severe cases. Take swabs for bacteriological examination first.

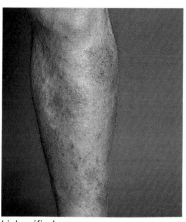

Lichenified eczema.

Dry, scaling, lichenified lesions
(1) Use emollients.
(2) Use steroid *ointments*, with antibiotics if infection is present.
(3) A weak coal tar preparation or ichthammol can be used on top of the ointments. This is particularly useful at night to prevent itching. 1–2% Coal tar can be prescribed in an ointment. For hard, lichenified skin salicylic acid can be incorporated and the following formulation has been found useful in our department:

● Coal tar solution *BP* 10%, salicylic acid 2%, and unguentum drench to 100%.
● 1% Ichthammol and 15% zinc oxide in white soft paraffin is less likely to irritate than tar and is suitable for children.

(4) In treating psoriasis start with a weaker tar preparation and progress to a stronger one.
(5) For thick, hyperkeratotic lesions, particulary in the scalp, salicylic acid is useful. It can be prescribed as 2–5% in aqueous cream, 1–2% in arachis oil, or 6% gel.

It is often easiest for the patient to apply the preparation to the scalp at night and wash it out the next morning with a tar shampoo.

Infection
Remember that secondary infection may be a cause of persisting lesions.

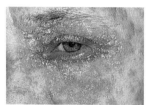 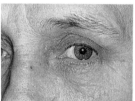

Infected eczema. Before and after treatment.

Hand dermatitis

Hand dermatitis: hints on management

(1) Hand washing:
Use tepid water and soap without perfume or colouring or chemicals added. Dry carefully, especially between fingers

(2) When in wet work:
Wear cotton gloves under rubber gloves (or plastic if you are allergic to rubber). Try not to use hot water and cut down to 15 minutes at a time if possible. Remove rings before wet or dry work. Use running water if possible

(3) Wear gloves in cold weather and for dusty work

(4) Use only ointments prescribed for you

(5) Things to avoid:
(a) Shampoo
(b) Peeling fruits and vegetables, especially citrus fruits
(c) Polishes of all kinds
(d) Solvents—e.g. white spirit, thinners, turpentine
(e) Hair lotions, creams, and dyes
(f) Detergents and strong cleansing agents
(g) "Unknown" chemicals

(6) Use "moisturisers" or emollients which have been recommended by your doctor—to counteract dryness

---

Hand dermatitis poses a particular problem in management and it is important that protection is continued after the initial rash has healed since it takes some time for the skin to recover its barrier function. Ointments or creams should be reapplied each time the hands have been washed.

It is useful to give patients a list of simple instructions such as those shown here.

Further reading
Atherton DJ. *Diet and children with eczema.* London: National Eczema Society, 1986.
Launer JM. *A practical guide to the management of eczema for general practitioners.* London: National Eczema Society, 1988.
Mackie RM. *Eczema and dermatitis.* London: Martin Dunitz, 1983.
Orton C. *Eczema relief: a complete guide to all remedies–alternative and orthodox.* London: Thorsons, 1990.

6. RASHES WITH EPIDERMAL CHANGES

| Lichen planus |
| Seborrhoeic dermatitis |

Pityriasis rosea
Pityriasis lichenoides
Localised lesions

Familiarity with the clinical features of psoriasis and eczema, which all clinicians see from time to time, provides a basis for comparison with other rather less common conditions.

The characteristics that each condition has in common with psoriasis and eczema are highlighted.

Lichen planus

Clinical features of psoriasis	Clinical features of eczema
Possible family history	Possible family history
Sometimes related to stress	Sometimes worse with stress
Itching—rare	Usually itching
Extensor surfaces and trunk	Flexor surfaces and face
Well defined, raised lesions	Poorly demarcated lesions
Hyperkeratosis	Oedema, vesicles, lichenification
Scaling, bleeding points beneath scales	Secondary infection sometimes present
Köebner's phenomenon	
Nails affected	
Scalp affected	
Mucous membranes not affected	

Like psoriasis, the lesions are well defined and raised. They also occur in areas of trauma—Koebner's phenomenon. There is no constant relation to stress. *Unlike* psoriasis, there is no family history. Itching is common. The distribution is on the flexor aspects of the limbs, particularly the ankles and wrists, rather than on the extensor surfaces, as in psoriasis. However, localised forms of lichen planus can occur on the shin, palm, and soles or elsewhere.

The typical flat topped lesions have a shiny hyperkeratotic lichenified surface with a violaceous colour, interrupted by milky white streaks—Wickham's striae. The oral mucosa is commonly affected with a white, net like appearance and sometimes ulceration.

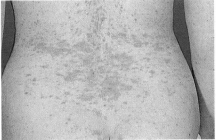
Lichen planus.

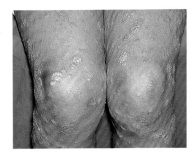
Lichen planus—legs

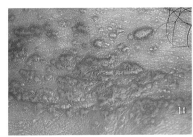
Lichen planus—skin.

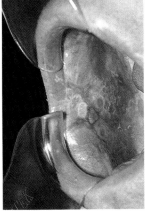
Lichen planus—oral mucosa.

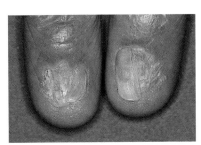
Lichen planus—nail.

Less commonly very thick hypertrophic lesions occur and also follicular lesions. Lichen planus is one cause of localised alopecia on the scalp as a result of hair follicle destruction.

Nail disease is less common than in psoriasis. There may be thinning and atrophy of part or all of a nail and these often take the form of a longitudinal groove.

Lichen planus usually resolves over many months to leave residual brown or grey macules. In the oral mucosa and areas subject to trauma ulceration can occur.

Rashes with epidermal changes

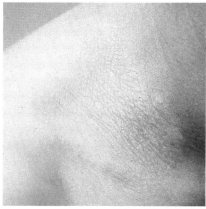

Lichenified eczema.

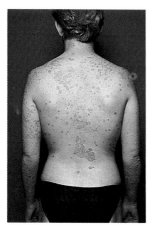

Guttate psoriasis.

Similar rashes

Lichenified eczema—This is also itchy and may occur on the ankles and wrists. The edge of the lesion is less well defined and is irregular. The flat topped, shiny papules are absent.

Guttate psoriasis is not as itchy as lichen planus. Scaling erythematous lesions do not have the lichenified surface of lichen planus.

Pityriasis lichenoides—The lesions have a mica like scale overlying an erythematous papule.

Drug eruptions—Rashes with many features of lichen planus can occur in patients taking:

Chloroquine ⎫
Chlorpropamide ⎬ The 3 "C"s
Chlorothiazide ⎭
Anti-inflammatory drugs
Gold preparations

It also occurs in those handling colour developers.

Treatment

The main symptom of itching is relieved to some extent by moderately potent steroid ointments. Very hypertrophic lesions may respond to strong steroid preparations under polythene occlusion. Careful intralesional injections may be very effective in persistent lesions. In very extensive, severe lichen planus systemic steroids may be indicated.

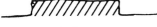

Guttate psoriasis.

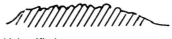

Lichenified eczema.

Lichen planus

Flexor surfaces
Mucous membranes affected
Itching common
Violaceous colour
Wickham's striae
Small discrete lesions
Lichenified

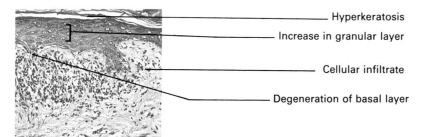

— Hyperkeratosis
— Increase in granular layer
— Cellular infiltrate
— Degeneration of basal layer

Pathology of lichen planus

As expected from the clinical appearance, there is hypertrophy and thickening of the epidermis with increased keratin. The white streaks seen clinically occur where there is pronounced thickness of the granular layer and underlying infiltrate. Degenerating basal cells may form "colloid bodies". The basal layer is being eaten away by an aggressive band of lymphocytes, the remaining papillae having a "saw toothed" appearance.

Seborrhoeic dermatitis

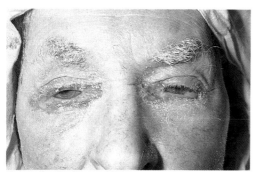

Seborrhoeic dermatitis.

Seborrhoeic dermatitis has nothing to do with sebum or any other kind of greasiness. There are two distinct types, adult and infantile.

Adult seborrhoeic dermatitis

The adult type is more common in men and in those with a tendency to scaling and dandruff in the scalp. There are several commonly affected areas:

(a) Seborrhoeic dermatitis affects the central part of the face, scalp, ears, and eyebrows. There may be an associated blepharitis, giving some red eyes and also otitis externa.

(b) The lesions over the sternum sometimes start as a single "medallion" lesion. A flower like "petaloid" pattern can occur. The back may be affected as well.

(c) Lesions also occur in well defined areas in the axillae and groin and beneath the breasts.

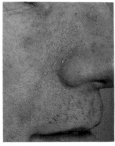

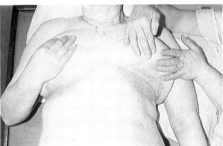

Seborrhoeic dermatitis.

Typically the lesions are discrete and erythematous and they may develop a yellow crust. The lesions tend to develop from the hair follicles. It is a persistent condition that varies in severity.

Clinically and pathologically the condition has features of both psoriasis and eczema. There is thickening of the epidermis with some of the inflammatory changes of psoriasis and the intercellular oedema of eczema. Parakeratosis—the presence of nuclei above the basement layer—may be noticeable. In recent years an increased number of *Pityrosporum ovale*, a normal commensal yeast, have been found.

Treatment—Topical steroids produce a rapid improvement, but not permanent clearing. Topical preparations containing salicylic acid, sulphur, or ichthammol may help in long term control. Triazole antifungal drugs by mouth have been reported to produce clearing and can be used topically. These drugs clear yeasts and fungi from the skin, including *P. ovale*, which is further evidence for the role of this organism.

Clinical features of psoriasis	Clinical features of eczema
Possible family history	Possible family history
Sometimes related to stress	Sometimes worse with stress
Itching—rare	Usually itching
Extensor surfaces and trunk	Flexor surfaces and face
Well defined, raised lesions	Poorly demarcated lesions
Hyperkeratosis	Oedema, vesicles, lichenification
Scaling, bleeding points beneath scales	Secondary infection sometimes present
Köebner's phenomenon	
Nails affected	
Scalp affected	
Mucous membranes not affected	

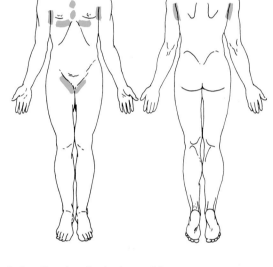

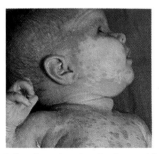

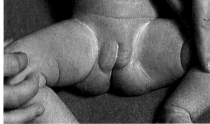

Infantile seborrhoeic dermatitis.

Infantile seborrhoeic dermatitis

In infants less than 6 months old a florid red eruption occurs with well defined lesions on the trunk and confluent areas in the flexures associated with scaling of the scalp. There is no consistent association with the adult type of seborrhoeic dermatitis. It has been suggested that infantile seborrhoeic dermatitis is a variant of atopic eczema. A high proportion of affected infants develop atopic eczema later but there are distinct differences. It is said to be more common in bottle fed infants.

Treatment comprises applying emollients, avoiding soap, and applying hydrocortisone combined with an antibiotic plus nystatin (for example, Terra-Cortril plus nystatin cream). Hydrocortisone can be used on the scalp.

Itching is present in atopic eczema but not in seborrhoeic dermatitis.

The clinical course of atopic eczema is prolonged with frequent exacerbations, whereas seborrhoeic dermatitis clears in a few weeks and seldom recurs.

Allergy—IgE concentrations are often raised in atopic eczema and food allergy is common, but not in seborrhoeic dermatitis.

Perioral dermatitis

Perioral dermatitis is possibly a variant of seborrhoeic dermatitis, with some features of acne. Papules and pustules develop around the mouth and chin. It occurs mainly in women.

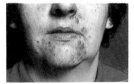

Perioral dermatitis.

Pityriasis rosea

Lichen planus
Seborrhoeic dermatitis

Pityriasis rosea
Pityriasis lichenoides
Localised lesions

The word "pityriasis" is from the Greek for bran, and the fine bran like scales on the surface are a characteristic feature. The numerous pale pink oval or round patches can be confused with psoriasis or discoid eczema. The history helps since this condition develops as an acute eruption and the patient can often point to a simple initial lesion—the herald patch.

There is commonly slight itching. Pityriasis rosea occurs mainly in the second and third decade, often during the winter months. "Clusters" of cases occur but not true epidemics. This suggests an infective basis. There may be prodromal symptoms with malaise, fever, or lymphadenopathy. Numerous causes have been suggested from allergy to fungi; the current favourite is a virus infection.

The typical patient is an adolescent or young adult, who is often more than a little concerned about the sudden appearance of a widespread rash. The lesions are widely distributed, often following skin creases, and concentrated on the trunk with scattered lesions on the limbs. The face and scalp may be affected.

Early lesions are red with fine scales—usually 1–4 cm in diameter. The initial herald patch is larger and may be confused with a fungal infection. Subsequently the widespread eruption develops in a matter of days or, rarely, weeks. As time goes by the lesions clear to give a slight pigmentation with a collarette of scales facing towards the centre.

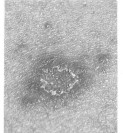 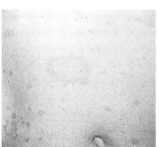 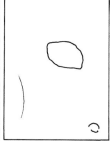

Herald lesions.

Clinical features of psoriasis	Clinical features of eczema
Possible family history	Possible family history
Sometimes related to stress	Sometimes worse with stress
Itching—rare	Usually itching
Extensor surfaces and trunk	Flexor surfaces and face
Well defined, raised lesions	Poorly demarcated lesions
Hyperkeratosis	Oedema, vesicles, lichenification
Scaling, bleeding points beneath scales	Secondary infection sometimes present
Köbner's phenomenon	
Nails affected	
Scalp affected	
Mucous membranes not affected	

Similar rashes

Discoid eczema presents with itching and lesions with erythema, oedema, and crusting rather than scaling. Vesicles may be present. The rash persists unchanged.

A *drug eruption* can sometimes produce similar lesions.

Guttate psoriasis—The lesions are more sharply defined and smaller (0·5–1·0 cm) and have waxy scales.

The pathology of pityriasis rosea

Histological changes are non-specific, showing slight inflammatory changes in the dermis, oedema, and slight hyperkeratosis.

Pityriasis lichenoides

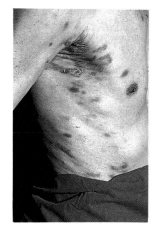

Pityriasis lichenoides is a less common condition occurring in acute and chronic forms.

The *acute* form presents with widespread pink papules which itch and form crusts, sometimes with vesicle formation suggestive of chickenpox. There may be ulceration. The lesions may develop in crops and resolve over a matter of weeks.

A mica scale pityrasis lichenoides.

The *chronic* form presents as reddish brown papules—often with a "mica" like scale that reveals a smooth, red surface underneath, unlike the bleeding points of psoriasis. In lichen planus there is no superficial scale and blistering is unusual.

The distribution is over the trunk, thighs, and arms, usually sparing the face and scalp.

The underlying pathology—vascular dilatation and a lymphocytic infiltrate with a keratotic scale—is in keeping with the clinical appearance. The cause is unknown. Treatment is with topical steroids.

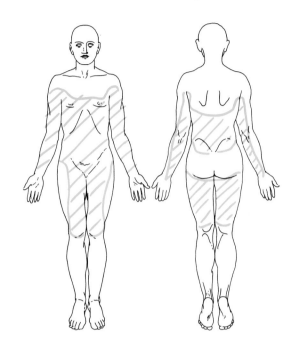

Clinical features of psoriasis	Clinical features of eczema
Possible family history	Possible family history
Sometimes related to stress	Sometimes worse with stress
Itching—rare	Usually itching
Extensor surfaces and trunk	Flexor surfaces and face
Well defined, raised lesions	Poorly demarcated lesions
Hyperkeratosis	Oedema, vesicles, lichenification
Scaling, bleeding points beneath scales	Secondary infection sometimes present
Köebner's phenomenon	
Nails affected	
Scalp affected	
Mucous membranes not affected	

Pityriasis versicolor

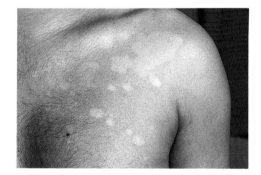

Pityriasis versicolor is a skin eruption that usually develops after sun exposure with white macules on the tanned skin but pale brown patches on the covered areas—hence the name—versicolor, or variable colour. The lesions are: (*a*) flat; (*b*) only *partially* depigmented—areas of vitiligo are totally white; and (*c*) do not show inflammation or vesicles.

The causitive organism is a yeast—*Pityrosporum orbiculare*—that takes advantage of some unknown change in the epidermis and develops a proliferative, stubby, mycelial form—*Malassezia furfur*. This otherwise incidental information can be simply put to practical use by taking a superficial scraping from a lesion on to a microscope slide—add a drop of potassium hydroxide or water with a coverslip. The organisms are readily seen under the microscope: spherical yeast forms and mycelial rods, resembling "grapes and bananas" ("spaghetti and meatballs" in the United States).

Treatment is simple: selenium sulphide shampoo applied regularly with ample water while showering or bathing will clear the infection. The colour change may take some time to clear. Ketoconazole shampoo is an effective alternative. Oral terbinafine, which is very effective in other fungal infections, has no effect.

Desquamating stage of generalised erythema

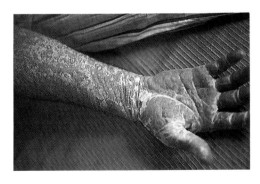

Any extensive acute erythema, from the erythroderma of psoriasis to a penicillin rash, commonly shows a stage of shedding large flakes of skin—desquamation—as it resolves. If only this stage is seen it can be confused with psoriasis.

Localised lesions with epidermal changes

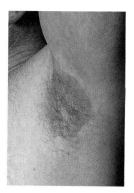

Flexural seborrhoeic dermatitis.

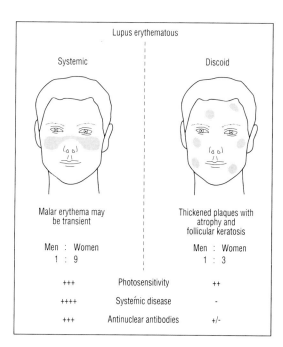

Corynebacterium minutissimum (erythrasma).

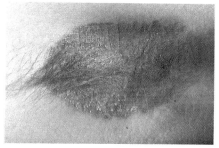

Lupus erythematous		
Systemic		Discoid
Malar erythema may be transient		Thickened plaques with atrophy and follicular keratosis
Men : Women 1 : 9		Men : Women 1 : 3
+++	Photosensitivity	++
++++	Systemic disease	-
+++	Antinuclear antibodies	+/-

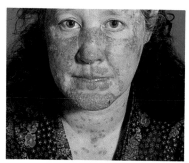

Systemic lupus erythematosus (subacute).

Psoriasis, seborrhoeic dermatitis, atopic eczema, and contact dermatitis can all present with localised lesions.

Psoriasis may affect only the flexures, occur as genital lesion, or affect only the palms. The lack of itching and epidermal changes with a sharp edge help in differentiation from infective or infiltrative lesions.

Seborrhoeic dermatitis can occur in the axillae or scalp with no lesions of other areas.

Atopic eczema—The "classical" sites in children—flexures of the elbows and knees and the face—may be modified to localised vesicular lesions on the hands and feet in older patients. Some atopic adults develop severe, persistent generalised eczematous changes.

Contact dermatitis is usually localised, by definition, to the areas in contact with irritant or allergen. Wide areas can be affected in reactions to clothing or washing powder, and sometimes the reaction extends beyond the site of contact.

Fungal infections—Apart from athlete's foot, toenail infections, and tinea cruris (most commonly in men) "ringworm" is in fact not as common as is supposed. The damp, soggy, itching skin of athlete's foot is well known. An itching, red diffuse rash in the groin differentiates tinea cruris from psoriasis. However, erythrasma, a bacterial infection, may be confused with seborrhoeic dermatitis and psoriasis—skin scrapings can be taken for culture of *Corynebacterium minutissimum* or, more simply, coral pink fluorescence shown with Wood's light. The scaling macules from dog and cat ringworm (*Microsporum canis*) itch greatly while the indurated pustular, boggy lesion (kerion) of cattle ringworm is quite distinctive.

Fungal infection of the axillae is rare; a red rash here is more likely to be due to erythrasma or seborrhoeic dermatitis.

Tinea cruris is very unusual before puberty and is uncommon in women.

In all cases of suspected fungal infection skin scrapings should be taken on to black paper, in which they can be folded and sent to the laboratory. In some units special "kits" are provided, which contain folded black paper and Sellotape strips on slides for taking a superficial layer of epidermis.

Lupus erythematosus—There are two forms of this condition: *discoid* (or DLE), which is usually limited to the skin, and *systemic* (or SLE), in which the skin lesions are associated with renal disease, arthritis, and other disorders. There is also a subacute type with limited systemic involvement.

Systemic lupus erythematosus, which is much more common in women than men, can be an acute, fulminating, multisystem disease that requires intensive treatment, or a more chronic progressive illness. Characteristically there is malar erythema with marked photosensitivity and a butterfly pattern. It may be transient. There may be scalp involvement as well with alopecia and also telangiectasia of the periungal blood vessels. Mouth ulcers may also be present.

Systemic involvement may cause nephritis, polyarteritis, leukopenia, pleurisy, myocarditis, and central nervous system involvement.

Systemic lupus erythematosis can present in many forms and immitate other diseases. The facial rash can resemble rosacea, cosmetic allergy or sun sensitivity. Systemic involvement may present with lassitude, weight loss, anaemia, arthritis, renal failure, dyspnoea, or cardiac signs, among others.

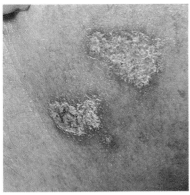

Discoid lupus erythematosus.

In discoid lupus erythematosus there are well-defined lesions with a combination of atrophy and hyperkeratosis of the hair follicles giving a "nutmeg grater" appearance. They occur predominantly on the cheeks, nose, and forehead. It is approximately three times as common in women as men, which is a lower ratio than in the systemic variety. There is a tendency for the skin lesions to gradually progress and to flare up on sun exposure. It is rare for progression to the systemic type to occur.

Treatment is with moderate to very potent topical steroids and hydroxychloroquine by mouth, together with suitable sun screens.

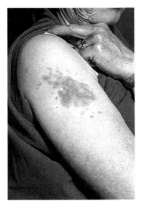

Fixed drug eruption.

Fixed drug eruptions—Generalised drug eruptions are considered under erythema, but there is a localised form recurring every time the drug is used. There is usually a well defined, erythematous plaque, sometimes with vesicles. Crusting, scaling, and pigmentation occur as the lesion heals. It is usually found on the limbs, and more than one lesion can occur.

Criteria for diagnosing systemic lupus erythematosus

Malar rash
Discoid plaques
Photosensitivity
Mouth ulcers
Arthritis
Serositis
Renal disease
Neurological disease
Haematological changes
Immunological changes
Anti nuclear antibodies

Criteria for making a diagnosis of SLE has been established of which at least four must be present.

In the subacute variety there is less severe systemic involvement, with scattered lesions occurring on the face, scalp, chest, and arms.

Systemic steroids are required for treatment with immunosuppressive agents if necessary. Antimalarial drugs, such as hydroxychloroquine, are more effective in the subacute type.

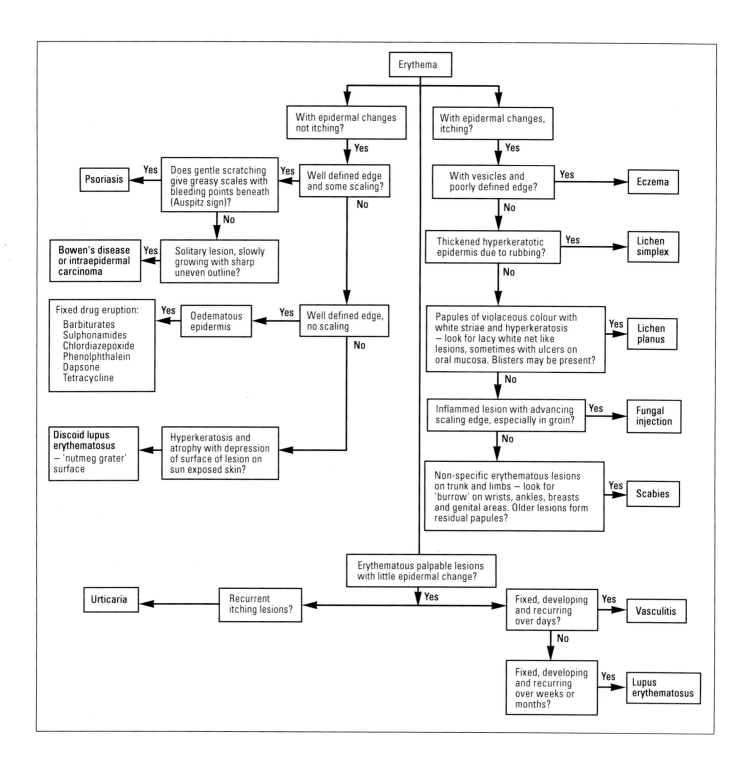

7. RASHES ARISING IN THE DERMIS

The erythemas

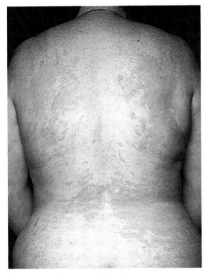

Erythema from antibiotics.

Complex reactions occurring in the capillaries and arterioles of the skin cause erythema— which is simply redness of the skin. This may present as flat macules or as papules, which are raised above the surrounding skin. The lesions may be transient or last for weeks, constant or variable in distribution, with or without vesicles.

It is possible to recognise specific patterns within this plethora of clinical signs, but even the most experienced dermatologist may be reduced to making a general diagnosis of "toxic" erythema. The best we can do therefore is to recognise the common types of erythema and list the possible causes. It is then a matter of deciding on the most likely underlying condition or group of conditions—for example, bacterial infection or autoimmune systemic disease.

Morphology and distribution

Because there can be the same cause for a variety of erythematous rashes detailed descriptions are of limited use. None the less, there are some characteristic patterns.

Morbilliform—The presentation of measles is well known, with the appearance of Koplik's spots on the mucosa, photophobia with conjunctivitis, and red macules behind the ears, spreading to the face, trunk, and limbs. The prodromal symptoms and conjunctivitis are absent in drug eruptions. Other viral conditions, including those caused by echoviruses, rubella, infectious mononucleosis, and erythema infectiosum may have to be considered.

Scarlatiniform rashes are similar to that in scarlet fever, when an acute erythematous eruption occurs in relation to a streptococcal infection. Characteristically erythema is widespread on the trunk. There is intense erythema and engorgement of the pharyngeal lymphoid tissue with an exudate and a "strawberry" tongue. Bacterial infections can produce a similar rash, as can drug rashes, without the systemic symptoms.

Figurate erythemas are chronic erythematous rashes forming annular or serpiginous patterns. There may be underlying malignancy or connective tissue disease.

Causes of "toxic" erythema

Drugs	antibiotics, barbiturates, thiazides
Infections	any recent infections such as streptococcal throat infection or erysipelas; spirochaetal infections; viral infections
Systemic causes	pregnancy; connective tissue disease; malignancy

---

Erythema multiforme

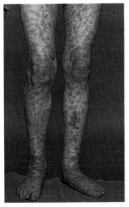 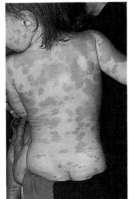

Erythema multiforme.

Erythema multiforme is sometimes misdiagnosed because of the variety of lesions and number of possible precipitating causes; some of these are listed below.

Infections	*Neoplasia*
Herpes simplex—the commonest cause	Hodgkin's disease
Mycoplasma infection	Myeloma
Infectious mononucleosis	Carcinoma
Poliomyelitis (vaccine)	*Chronic inflammation*
Many other viral and bacterial infections	Sarcoidosis
Any focal sepsis	Wegener's granuloma
BCG inoculaton	*Drugs*
Collagen disease	Barbiturates
Systemic lupus erythematosus	Sulphonamides
Polyarteritis nodosa	Penicillin
	Phenothiazine and many others

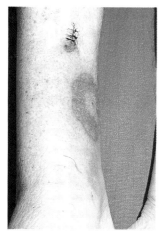

Annular lesions of erythema multiforme.

Clinical picture

The usual erythematous lesions occur in crops on the limbs and trunk. Each lesion may extend, leaving a cyanotic centre, which produces an "iris" or "target" lesion. Bullae may develop in the lesions and on the mucous membranes. A severe bullous form, with lesions on the mucous membranes, is known as the Stevens-Johnson syndrome. There may be neural and bronchial changes as well. Barbiturates, sulphonamides, and other drugs are the most common cause.

Histologically there are inflammatory changes, vasodilatation, and degeneration of the epidermis.

A condition that may be confused is *Sweet's syndrome*, which presents as acute plum coloured raised painful lesions on the limbs—sometimes the face and neck—with fever. It is more common in women. The alternative name, "acute febrile neutrophilic dermatosis," describes the presentation and the pathological findings of a florid neutrophilic infiltrate. There is often a preceding upper respiratory infection. Treatment with steroids produces a rapid response but recurrences are common.

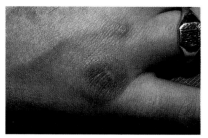

Annular lesions of erythema multiforme.

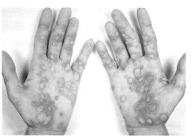

Blistering lesions.

Erythema induratum

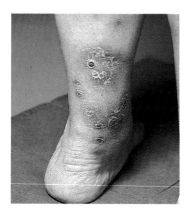

Erythema induratum occurs on the lower legs posteriorly, usually in women, with diffuse, indurated dusky red lesions that may ulcerate. It is more common in patients with poor cutaneous circulation. Epithelioid cell granulomas may form.

It was originally described in association with tuberculous infection elsewhere in the body (Bazin's disease). It represents a vasculitic reaction to the infection, and when there is no tuberculous infection another chronic infection may be responsible.

Erythema nodosum

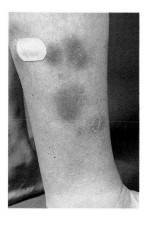

Erythema nodosum occurs as firm, gradually developing lesions, predominantly on the extensor aspect of the legs. They are tender and progress from an acute erythematous stage to residual lesions resembling bruises over four to eight weeks.

Single or multiple lesions occur varying in size from 1 to 5 cm. The lesions are often preceded by an upper respiratory tract infection and may be associated with fever and arthralgia. Infections (streptococcal, tuberculous, viral, and fungal) and sarcoidosis are the commonest underlying conditions. Drugs can precipitate erythema nodosum, the contraceptive pill and the sulphonamides being the commonest cause. Ulcerative colitis, Crohn's disease, and lymphoma may also be associated with the condition.

Rashes due to drugs

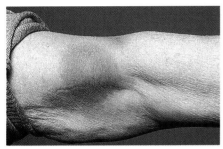

Fixed drug eruption.

There is an almost infinite variety of types of drug reaction.

External contact with drugs can cause a contact dermatitis presenting with eczematous changes. This occurs commonly with neomycin and bacitracin. Chloramphenicol and sulphonamides from ophthalmic preparations can also cause dermatitis around the eyes. Penicillin is a potent sensitiser so is not used for topical treatment.

Drugs used *systemically* can cause a localised fixed drug eruption or a more diffuse macular or papular erythema, symmetrically distributed. In the later stages exfoliation, with shedding scales of skin, may develop. Antibiotics, particularly penicillins, are the most common cause. They also cause erythema multiforme as already mentioned.

Penicillins are the most common cause of drug rashes, which range from acute anaphylaxis to persistent diffuse erythematous lesions. Joint pains, fever, and proteinuria may be associated, as in serum sickness.

Ampicillin often produces a characteristic erythematous maculopapular rash on the limbs 7–20 days after the start of treatment. Such rashes occur in nearly all patients with infectious mononucleosis who are given ampicillin.

Other reactions

Blistering eruptions	Barbiturates
	Sulphonamides
	Iodines/bromides
	Chlorpropamide
	Salicylates
	Phenylbutazone
Lichen planus like reactions	Chloroquine
	Chlorothiazide
	Chlorpropamide
Photosensitivity (seen on areas exposed to light)	Thiazide diuretics
	Sulphonamides
	Tetracyclines

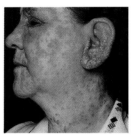

Topical neomycin allergy.

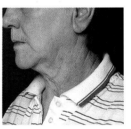

After withdrawing neomycin.

Vasculitis

Vasculitis

Inflammation around dilated capillaries and small blood vessels:

- a common component of the erythemas
- may occur as red macules and papules with necrotic lesions on the extremities
- in children a purpuric type (Henoch–Schönlein purpura) occurs in association with nephritis
- systemic lesions may occur, with renal, joint, gastrointestinal, and central nervous system involvement

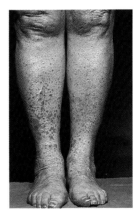

Inflammation associated with immune complexes in the capillaries and small blood vessels is part of the pathological changes of many of the conditions described above. The term vasculitis is also used clinically to describe a variable clinical picture with red macules and papules and with necrosis and bruising in severe cases. In children purpura is more prominent and these cases are classified as Henoch–Schönlein purpura. The legs and arms are usually affected. Skin signs are preceded by malaise and fever with arthropathy and there may be associated urticaria. Since a high proportion of cases are associated with systemic lesions it is essential to check for renal, joint, gastrointestinal, and central nervous system disease. In children with Henoch–Schönlein purpura nephritis is common.

Purpura

Is seen on the skin as a result of:

- thrombocytopenia—platelet deficiency
- senile purpura—due to shearing of capillaries as a result of defective supporting connective tissue
- purpura in patients on corticosteroid treatment—similar to senile purpura
- Schamberg's disease—brown macules and red spots resembling cayenne pepper on the legs of men
- associated vasculitis

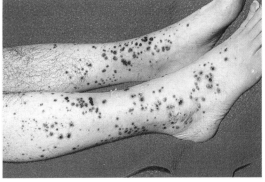
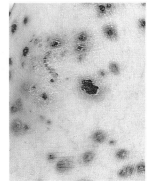

Acute vasculitis with necrosis.

Some conditions associated with vasculitis

Infection—streptococcal, hepatitis

Drugs—numerous, including sulphonamides, penicillin, phenothiazine, phenacitin

Chemicals—insecticides, weed killers, phenolic compounds

Connective tissue diseases—systemic lupus erythematosus, rheumatoid arthritis

Lymphoma and leukaemia

Dysproteinaemias

Urticaria

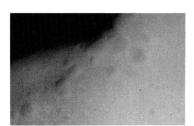

Urticaria.

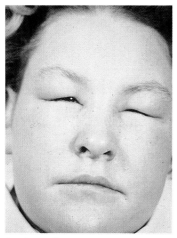

Angio-oedema.

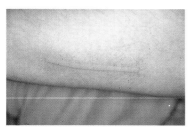

Dermatographism.

In this condition itching red weals develop; they resemble the effects of stinging nettle (*Urtica dioica*) on the skin. The condition may be associated with allergic reactions, infection, or physical stimuli, but in most patients no cause can be found. Similar lesions may precede, or be associated with, vasculitis (*urticarial vasculitis*), pemphigoid, or dermatitis herpetiformis.

The histological changes may be very slight but usually there is oedema, vasodilation, and a cellular infiltrate of lymphocytes, polymorphs, and histiocytes. Various vasoactive substances are thought to be involved, including histamine, kinins, leukotrienes, prostaglandins, and complement.

Angio-oedema is due to oedema of the subcutaneous tissues; it can occur rapidly and may involve the mucous membranes. *Hereditary angio-oedema* is a rare form with recurrent severe episodes of subcutaneous oedema, swelling of the mucous membranes, and systemic symptoms. Laryngeal oedema is the most serious complication.

The physical urticarias, which account for about 25% of cases, include *dermatographism* and the *pressure, cold, heat, solar, cholinergic*, and *aquagenic urticarias*.

Dermatographism is an exaggerated release of histamine from stroking the skin firmly with a hard object, such as the end of a pencil. *Pressure urticaria* is caused by sustained pressure from clothing, hard seats, and footwear; it may last some hours. *Cold urticaria* varies in severity and is induced by cold, particulary by cold winds or by the severe shock of bathing in cold water. It appears early in life—in infancy in the rare familial form. In a few cases abnormal serum proteins may be found. *Heat urticaria* is rare, but warm environments often make physical urticaria worse. *Solar urticaria* is a rare condition in which sunlight causes an acute urticarial eruption. Tolerance to sun exposure may develop in areas of the body normally exposed to sun. There is sensitivity to a wide spectrum of ultraviolet light. *Cholinergic urticaria* is characterised by the onset of itching urticarial papules after exertion, stress, or exposure to heat. The injection of cholinergic drugs induces similar lesions in some patients. *Aquagenic urticaria* occurs on contact with water, regardless of the temperature.

Non-physical urticaria may be *acute* in association with allergic reactions to insect bites, drugs, and other factors. Chronic recurrent urticaria is fairly common. Innumerable causes have been suggested but, to the frustration of patient and doctor alike, it is often impossible to identify any specific factor. Some reported causes are listed below.

Some reported causes of non-physical urticaria

Food allergies—fish, eggs, dairy products, chocolate, nuts, strawberries, pork, tomatoes

Food additives—e.g. tartrazine dyes, sodium benzoates

Salicylates—both in medicines and foods

Infection—bacterial, viral, and protozoal

Systemic disorders—autoimmune and "collagen" diseases; reticuloses, carcinoma, and dysproteinaemias

Contact urticaria—may occur from contact with meat, fish, vegetables, plants, and animals, among many other factors

Papular urticaria—a term used for persistent itching papules at the site of insect bites; it is also sometimes applied to urticaria from other causes

Inhalants—e.g. house dust, animal danders

Treatment

(1) Eliminate possible causative factors, such as aspirin, and by a diet free from food additives

(2) Antihistamines. Also, H_2 blockers—e.g. cimetidine

(3) Adrenaline can be used for acute attacks, particularly if there is angio-oedema of the respiratory tract

(4) Systemic corticosteroids should not be used for chronic urticaria but may be needed for acute urticarial vasculitis

Further reading

Berlit P, Moore P. *Vasculitis, rheumatic diseases and the nervous system.* Berlin: Springer-Verlag, 1992.
Champion RH, Greaves MW, Black AK. *The urticarias.* Edinburgh: Churchill Livingstone, 1985.
Czarnetzki BM. *Urticaria.* Berlin: Springer-Verlag, 1986.

8. BLISTERS AND PUSTULES

Development, duration, and distribution

<table>
<tr><td>

The differential diagnosis of blistering eruptions

Widespread blisters

Eczema—lichenfication and crusting, itching

Dermatitis herpetiformis—itching, extensor surface, persistent

Chickenpox—crops of blisters, self limiting, prodromal illness

Pityriasis lichenoides—pink papules, developing blisters

Erythema multiforme—erythematous and "target" lesions, mucous membranes affected

Pemphigoid—older patients, trunk and flexures affected. Preceding erythematous lesions, deeply situated, tense blisters

Pemphigus—adults, widespread superficial blisters, mucous membranes affected (erosions)

Drug eruptions—history of drugs prescribed, overdose (barbiturates, tranquillisers)

Localised blisters

Eczema—"pompholyx" blisters on hand and feet, itching

Allergic reactions, including topical medication, insect bites

Psoriasis—deep, sterile, non-itching blisters on palms and soles

Impetigo—usually localised, staphylococci and streptococci isolated

Herpes simplex—itching lesions developing turbid blisters

</td></tr>
</table>

Itching	Non-itching	
Eczema-pompholyx on hands and feet	Erythema multiforme	Pustular psoriasis of hands and feet
Allergic reactions	Pemphigus vulgaris	
Dermatitis herpetiformis	Bullous pemphigoid	
Chickenpox	Bullous impetigo	
Herpes simplex	Insect bite allergy	

Several diseases may present with blisters or pustules. There is no common condition that can be used as a "reference point" with which less usual lesions can be compared in the same way as rashes can be compared with psoriasis. A different approach is needed for the assessment of blistering or pustular lesions, based on the history and appearance and summarised as the three Ds: development, duration, and distribution.

Development—Was there any preceding systemic illness—as in chickenpox, hand, foot, and mouth disease, and other viral infections? Was there a preceding area of erythema—as in herpes simplex or pemphigoid? Is the appearance of the lesions associated with itching—as in herpes simplex, dermatitis herpetiformis, and eczematous vesicles on the hands and feet?

Duration—Some acute blistering arises rapidly—for example, in allergic reactions, impetigo, erythema multiforme, and pemphigus. Other blisters have a more gradual onset and follow a chronic course—as in dermatitis herpetiformis, pityriasis lichenoides, and the bullae of porphyria cutanea tarda. The rare genetic disorder epidermolysis bullosa is present from, or soon after, birth.

Distribution—The distribution of blistering rashes helps considerably in making a clinical diagnosis. The most common patterns of those that have a fairly constant distribution are shown.

Itching is a very useful symptom. If all the accessible lesions are scratched and it is hard to find an intact blister it is probably an itching rash.

Clinical features: widespread blisters

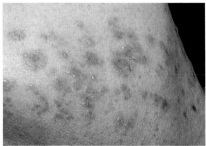

Dermatitis herpetiformis.

Chickenpox

Chickenpox is so well known in general practice that it is rarely seen in hospital clinics and is sometimes not recognised. The prodromal illness lasts one to two days and is followed by erythematous lesions that rapidly develop vesicles, then pustules, followed by crusts in two to three days. Crops of lesions develop at the same sites—usually on the trunk, face, scalp, and limbs. The oral mucosa may be affected. The condition is usually benign.

Dermatitis herpetiformis

Dermatitis herpetiformis occurs in early and middle adult life and is characterised by symmetrical, intensely itching vesicles on the trunk

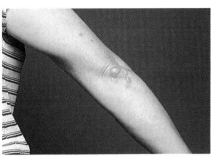

Dermatitis herpetiformis.

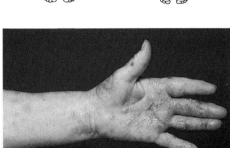

Erythema multiforme.

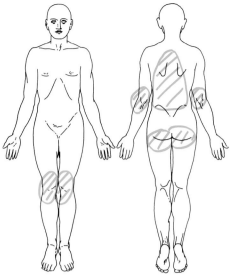

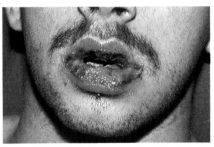

Pityriasis lichenoides.

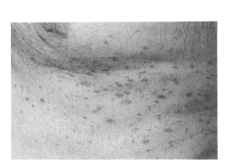

Bullous pemphigoid.

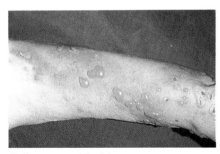

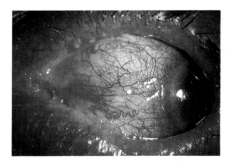

Mucous membrane pemphigoid.

and extensor surfaces. The vesicles are superficial. The onset is gradual, but may occur rapidly. The distribution is shown in the diagram.

Variants of dematitis herpetiformis are larger blisters forming bullae and erythematous papules and vesicles.

Associated conditions—Coeliac disease with villous atrophy and gluten intolerance may occur in association with dermatitis herpetiformis. Linear IgA disease is a more severe, widespread disease, in which there are "linear" deposits of IgA along the basement membrane of the epidermis and not only at the tips of the papillae as in dermatitis herpetiformis. Treatment is with dapsone or sulphapyridine together with a gluten free diet.

Erythema multiforme with blisters

Blisters can occur on the lesions of erythema multiforme to a variable degree; when severe, generalised, and affecting the mucous membranes it is known as Stevens–Johnson syndrome. The typical erythematous maculopapular changes develop over one to two days with a large blister (bulla) developing in the centre of the target lesions. In severe progressive cases there is extensive disease of the mouth, eyes, genitalia, and respiratory tract. The blisters are subepidermal—that is, deep— although some basement membrane remains on the floor of the blister.

Pityriasis lichenoides varioliformis acuta

As the name implies lichenified papules are the main feature of pityriasis lichenoides varioliformis acuta (or Mucha-Habermann's disease), but vesicles occur in the acute form. Crops of pink papules develop centrally, with vesicles, necrosis, and scales—resembling those of chickenpox, hence the "varioliformis". There is considerable variation in the clinical picture, and a prodromal illness may occur. The condition may last from six weeks to six months. No infective agent has been isolated. The pathological changes parallel the clinical appearance with inflammation around the blood vessels and oedema within the dermis.

Pemphigoid

The bullous type of pemphigoid is a disease of the elderly in which tense bullae develop rapidly, often over a preceding erythematous rash, as well as on normal skin. The flexuaral aspects of the limbs and trunk are mainly affected. The bullae are subepidermal and persistent, with antibodies deposited at the dermoepidermal junction. Unlike pemphigus, there is a tendency for the condition to remit after many months. Treatment is with corticosteroids by mouth, 40–60 mg daily in most patients, although higher doses are required by some. Azathioprine aids remission, with reduced steroid requirements, but takes some weeks to produce an effect. Topical steroids can be used on developing lesions.

Chronic scarring pemphigoid affects the mucous membranes with small bullae that break down, leading to erosions and adhesions in the conjunctivae, mouth, pharynx, and genitalia.

There is also a localised type of pemphigoid occurring on the legs of elderly women that runs a benign self limiting course.

Blisters and pustules

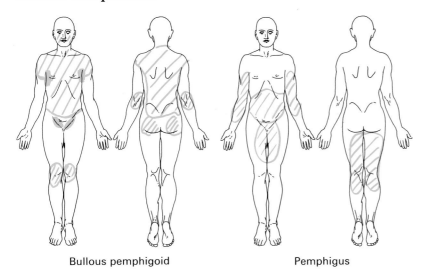

Bullous pemphigoid   Pemphigus

Pemphigus

The most common form of pemphigus vulgaris is a chronic progressive condition with widespread superficial bullae arising in normal skin. In about half of the cases this is preceded by blisters and erosions in the mouth. The bullae are easily broken, and even rubbing apparently normal skin causes the superficial epidermis to slough off (Nikolsky sign). These changes are associated with the deposition of immunoglobulin in the epidermal intercellular spaces. It is a serious condition with high morbidity despite treatment with steroids and azathioprine.

Pemphigus vegetans and pemphigus erythematosus are less common variants.

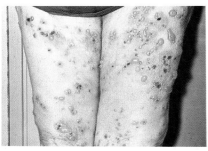

Pemphigus vulgaris.

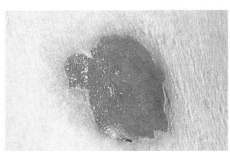

Nikolsky sign.

Differential diagnosis of ulcers in the mouth

Trauma (dentures)

Aphthous ulcers

Candida albicans infection

Herpes simplex

Erythema multiforme (from drugs)

Pemphigus

Lichen planus

Carcinoma

Clinical features: localised blisters

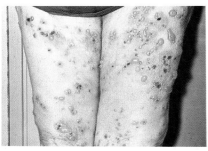

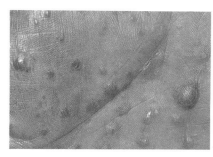

Pompholyx—which means "a bubble"—is characterised by persistent, itchy, clear blisters on the fingers, which may extend to the palms, with larger blisters. The feet may be affected. Secondary infection leads to turbid vesicle fluid. Pompholyx may be associated with a number of conditions—atopy, stress, fungal infection elsewhere, and allergic reactions. It may occur as a result of ingesting nickel in nickel sensitive patients and a similar reaction has been reported to neomycin.

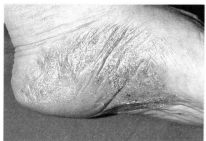

Pustular psoriasis is characterised by deep seated sterile blisters, often with no sign of psoriasis elsewhere—hence the term *palmopustular pustulosis*. Foci of sepsis have long been considered a causative factor and recent studies have shown a definite association with cigarette smoking. The pattern of HLA antigens indicates that this may be a separate condition from psoriasis.

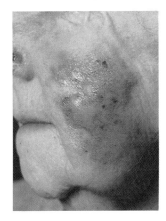

Bullous impetigo is seen in children and adults. Staphylococci are usually isolated from the blister fluid. The blisters are commonly seen on the face and are more deeply situated than in the non-bullous variety.

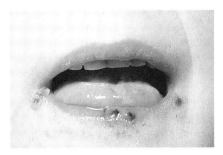

Herpes simplex—Primary infection with type I virus occurs on the face, lips, and buccal mucosa in children and young adults. Type II viruses cause genital infection. Itching may be severe.

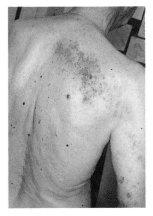

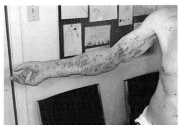

Herpes zoster is due to varicella virus producing groups of vesicles in a dermatome distribution, usually thoracic, trigeminal, or lumbosacral. It is more common after the fourth decade of life.

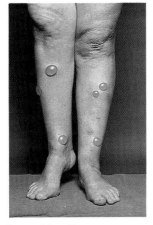

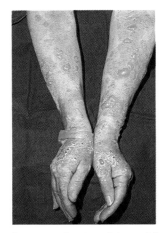

Insect bite allergy—Large blisters, which are usually not itching, can occur on the legs of susceptible individuals.

Bullous drug eruptions

Fixed drug eruptions can develop bullae, and some drugs can cause a generalised bullous eruption, particularly:

Barbiturates (particularly if taken in overdosage)
Sulphonamides
Penicillamine (captopril, penicillins (which produce pemphigus-like bullae))
Frusemide (may be phototoxic)

Remember that there may be an associated erythematous eruption.

Insect bite allergy.　　　　Drug reaction to sulphapyridine.

41

9. LEG ULCERS

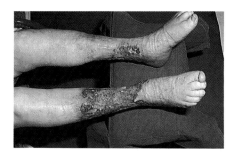

Although the patient will not probably die of this disease, yet, without great care, it may render her miserable. The disease may be very much relieved by art, and it is one of very common occurrence.

SIR BENJAMIN BRODIE (1846)

Despite the great increase in our understanding of the pathology of leg ulcers, their management is still largely "art". Consequently there are numerous treatments, each with their enthusiastic advocates. There are, however, basic concepts which are helpful in management. Since about 95% of leg ulcers are of the "venous" or gravitational variety these will be considered first.

Pathology of venous ulcers

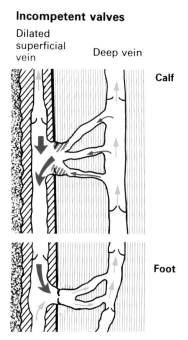

Healthy

Superficial vein | Deep vein
Calf

Skin | Rigid fascia | Muscle "pump"

Subcutaneous tissue

Incompetent valves

Dilated superficial vein | Deep vein
Calf

Foot

The skin—Ulcers arise because the skin dies from inadequate provision of nutrients and oxygen. This occurs as a consequence of (*a*) oedema in the subcutaneous tissues with poor lymphatic and capillary drainage; and (*b*) the extravascular accumulation of fibrinous material that has leaked from the blood vessels. The result is a rigid cuff around the capillaries, preventing diffusion through the wall, and fibrosis of the surrounding tissues.

The blood vessels—Arterial perfusion of the leg is usually normal or increased, but stasis occurs in the venules. The lack of venous drainage is a consquence of incompetent valves between the superficial veins and the deeper large veins on which the calf muscle "pump" acts. In the normal leg there is a *superficial* low pressure venous system and *deep* high pressure veins. If the blood flow from superficial to deep veins is reversed then the pressure in the superficial veins may increase to a level that prevents venous drainage with "back pressure" causing stasis and oedema.

Incompetent valves leading to gravitational ulcers may be preceded by:
(*a*) deep vein thrombosis associated with pregnancy or, less commonly, leg injury, immobilisation, or infarctions in the past;
(*b*) primary long saphenous vein insufficiency;
(*c*) familial venous valve incompetence that presents at an earlier stage. There is a familial predisposition in half of all patients with leg ulcers; or
(*d*) deep venous obstruction.

Who gets ulcers?
Mainly women get ulcers—2% of those over 80 having venous ulcers as a long term consequence of the factors listed above. Leg ulcers are more likely to occur and are more severe in obese people.

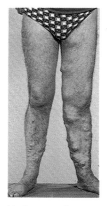
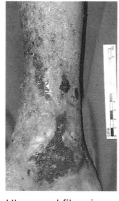

Varicose veins.   Ulcers and fibrosis.

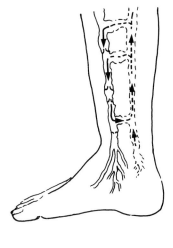

Clinical changes

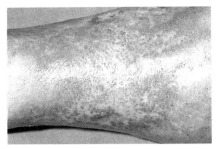

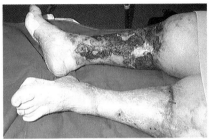

Atrophie blanche.

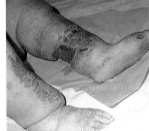

Champagne bottle legs.

Oedema and fibrinous exudate often lead to fibrosis of the subcutaneous tissues, which may be associated with localised loss of pigment and dilated capillary loops, an appearance known as "atrophie blanche". This occurs around the ankle with oedema and dilated tortuous superficial veins proximally and can lead to "champagne bottle legs", the bottle, of course, being inverted. Ulceration often occurs for the first time after a trivial injury.

Lymphoedema results from obliteration of the superficial lymphatics, with associated fibrosis. There is often hypertrophy of the overlying epidermis with a "polypoid" appearance, also known as lipodermatosclerosis.

Venous ulcers occur around the ankles, commonly over the medial malleolus. The margin is usually well defined with a shelving edge, and a slough may be present. There may also be surrounding eczematous changes. Venous ulcers are not usually painful but arterial ulcers are.

It is important to check the pulses in the leg and foot as compression bandaging of a leg with impaired blood flow can cause ischaemia and necrosis.

Treatment

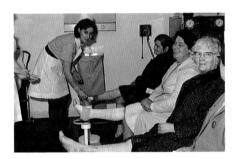

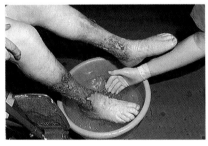

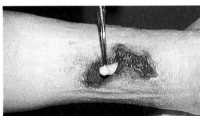

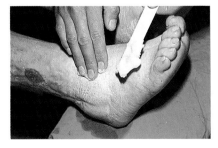

When new epidermis can grow across an ulcer it will and the aim is to produce an environment in which this can take place. To this end several measures can be taken.

(1) *Oedema* may be reduced by means of (*a*) diuretics, (*b*) keeping the legs elevated when sitting, (*c*) avoiding standing as far as possible. Raising the heels slightly from time to time helps venous return by the "calf muscle pump", (*d*) applying compression bandages, which may do more harm than good *unless* they are applied *before* the patient gets out of bed in the morning, when there is minimal oedema, and applied with more pressure on the foot than the calf, so as to create a pressure gradient towards the thigh.

(2) *Exudate and slough* should be removed. Lotions can be used to clean the ulcer and as compresses—0·9% saline solution, sodium hypochlorite solution, Eusol, or 5% hydrogen peroxide.

There is some evidence that antiseptic solutions and chlorinated solutions (such as sodium hypochlorite and Eusol) delay collagen production and cause inflammation. Enzyme preparations may help by "digesting" the slough. To prevent the formation of granulation tissue use silver nitrate 0·25% compresses, a silver nitrate "stick" for more exuberant tissue, and curettage, if necessary.

(3) *The dressings* applied to the ulcer can consist of (*a*) simple non-stick, paraffin gauze dressings. An allergy may develop to those with an antibiotic; (*b*) wet compresses with saline or silver nitrate solutions for exudative lesions; (*c*) silver sulphadiazine (Flamazine) or hydrogen peroxide creams (Hioxyl); and (*d*) absorbent dressings, consisting of hydrocolloid patches or powder, which are helpful for smaller ulcers.

(4) *Paste bandages*, impregnated with zinc oxide and antiseptics or ichthammol, help to keep dressings in place and provide protection. They may, however, traumatise the skin, and allergic reactions to their constituents are not uncommon.

(5) *Treatment of infection* is less often necessary than is commonly supposed. All ulcers are colonised by bacteria to some extent, usually coincidental staphylococci. A purulent exudate is an indication for a broad spectrum antibiotic and a swab for bacteriology. Erythema, oedema, and tenderness around the ulcers suggest a β haemolytic streptococcal infection, which will require long term antibiotic treatment. Dyes can be painted on the edge of the ulcer, where they fix to the bacterial wall as well as the patient's skin. In Scotland bright red eosin is traditionally used, while in the south a blue dye, gentian violet, is favoured.

Systemic antibiotics have little effect on ulcers but are indicated if there is surrounding cellulitis. A swab for culture and sensitivity helps to keep track of organisms colonising the area.

Leg ulcers

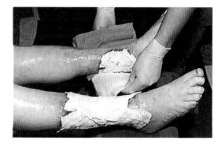

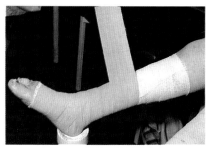

(6) *Surrounding eczematous changes* should be treated. Use topical steroids, not more than medium strength, avoiding the ulcer itself. Ichthammol 1% in 15% zinc oxide and white soft paraffin or Ichthopaste bandages can be used as a protective layer, and topical antibiotics can be used if necessary. It is important to remember that any of the commonly used topical preparations can cause an allergic reaction: neomycin, lanolin, formaldehyde, tars, Chinaform (the "C" of many proprietary steroids).

(7) *Skin grafting* can be very effective. There must be a healthy viable base for the graft, with an adequate blood supply; natural re-epithelialisation from the edges of the ulcer is a good indication that a graft will be supported. Pinch grafts or partial thickness grafts can be used. Any clinical infection, particularly with pseudomonal organisms, should be treated.

(8) *Maintaining general health*, with adequate nutrition and weight reduction, is important.

(9) *Corrective surgery* for associated venous abnormalities.

In treating venous leg ulcers

(1) Take measures to eliminate oedema and reduce weight—make sure the patient understands these

(2) Never apply steroid preparations to the ulcer itself or it will not heal. Make sure that both nurses and patients are aware of this

(3) Beware of allergy developing to topical agents—especially to antibiotics

(4) There is no need to submit the patient to a variety of antibiotics according to the differing bacteria isolated from leg ulcer slough, unless there is definite evidence of infection of adjacent tissue clinically

(5) A vascular "flare" around the ankle and heel with varicose veins, sclerosis, or oedema indicates a high risk of ulceration developing

(6) Make sure arterial pulses are present. A Doppler apparatus can be used

---

Arterial ulcers

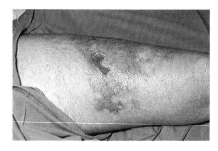

Ulcers on the leg also occur as a result of (*a*) atherosclerosis with poor peripheral circulation, particularly in older patients; (*b*) vasculitis affecting the larger subcutaneous arteries; and (*c*) aterial obstruction in macroglobulinaemia, cryoglobulinaemia, polycythaemia, and "collagen" disease—particularly rheumatoid arthritis.

Arterial ulcers are sharply defined and accompanied by pain, which may be very severe, especially at night. The leg, especially the pretibial area, is affected rather than the ankle. In patients with hypertension a very tender ulcer can develop posteriorly (Martorelli's ulcer).

As mentioned above, compression bandaging will make arterial ulcers worse and may lead to ischaemia of the leg.

Diagnosis

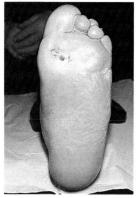

Ulcer in diabetic foot.

The differing presentation of arterial and venous ulcers helps in distinguishing between them, but some degree of aterial insufficiency often complicates venous ulcers.

Phlebography and Doppler ultrasound may help in detecting venous incompetence and arterial obstruction, which can sometimes be treated surgically.

Ulcers on the leg may also occur secondary to other diseases, because of infection, in malignant disease, and after trauma.

Secondary ulcers—Ulcers occur in diabetes, in periarteritis nodosa, and in vasculitis. Pyoderma gangrenosum, a chronic necrotic ulcer with surrounding induration, may occur in association with ulcerative colitis or rheumatoid vasculitis.

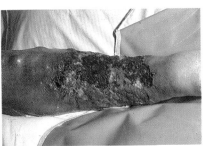

Squamous cell carcinoma in venous ulcer.

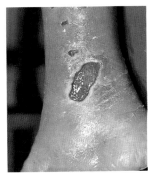

Tuberculous ulceration.

Infections that cause ulcers include staphylococcal or streptococcal infections, tuberculosis (which is rare in the United Kingdom but may be seen in recent immigrants), and anthrax.

Malignant diseases—Squamous cell carcinoma may present as an ulcer or, rarely, develop in a pre-existing ulcer. Basal cell carcinoma and melanoma may develop into ulcers, as may Kaposi's sarcoma.

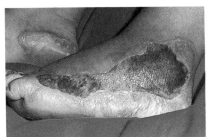

Dermatitis artefacta.

Trauma—Patients with diabetic or other types of neuropathy are at risk of developing trophic ulcers. Rarely they may be self induced—"dermatitis artefacta".

Further reading

Browse NL, Burnand KG, Lea TM. *Diseases of the veins: pathology, diagnosis and treatment.* London: Edward Arnold, 1988.
Kappert A. *Diagnosis of peripheral vascular disease.* Berne: Hauber, 1971.
Ryan TJ. *The management of leg ulcers.* 2nd ed. Oxford: Oxford University Press, 1987.

10. ACNE AND ROSACEA

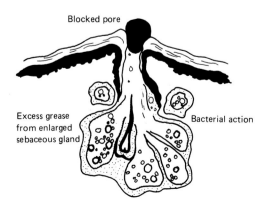

Acne goes with adolescence, a term derived from the Greek "acme" or prime of life. The young girl who is desperately aware of the smallest comedo and the young man, with his face or back a battle field of acne cysts and scars, are familiar to us all. Both need treatment and help in coming to terms with their condition.

What is acne?

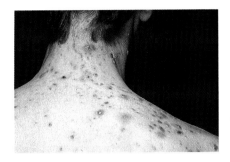

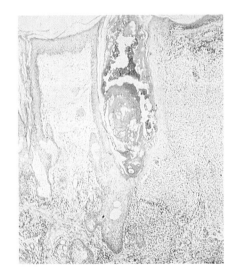

Blocked pore

Excess grease from enlarged sebaceous gland

Bacterial action

Acne lesions develop from the sebaceous glands associated with hair follicles—on the face, external auditory meatus, back, chest, and anogenital area. (Sebaceous glands are also found on the eyelids and mucosa, prepuce and cervix, where they are not associated with hair follicles.) The sebaceous gland contains holocrine cells that secrete triglycerides, fatty acids, wax esters, and sterols as "sebum". The main changes in acne are:

(a) an increase in sebum secretion;

(b) thickening of the keratin lining of the sebaceous duct, to produce blackheads or comedones. The colour of blackheads is due to melanin, not dirt;

(c) an increase in *Propionibacterium acnes* bacteria in the duct;

(d) an increase in free fatty acids;

(e) inflammation around the sebaceous gland; probably as a result of the release of bacterial enzymes.

Underlying causes

There are various underlying causes of these changes.

Hormones—Androgenic hormones increase the size of sebaceous glands and the amount of sebum in both male and female adolescents. Oestrogens have the opposite effect in prepubertal boys and eunuchs. In some women with acne there is lowering of the concentration of sex hormone binding globulin and a consequent increase in free testosterone concentrations. There is probably also a variable increase in androgen sensitivity. Oral contraceptives containing more than 50 µg ethinyloestradiol can make acne worse and the combined type may lower sex hormone binding globulin concentrations, leading to increased free testosterone. Infantile acne occurs in the first few months of life and may last some years. Apart from rare causes, such as adrenal hyperplasia or virilising tumours, transplacental simulation of the adrenal gland is thought to result in the release of adrenal androgens—but this does not explain why the lesions persist. It is more common in boys.

Fluid retention—The premenstrual exacerbation of acne is thought to be due to fluid retention leading to increased hydration of and swelling of the duct. Sweating also makes acne worse, possibly by the same mechanism.

Diet—in some patients acne is made worse by chocolate, nuts, and coffee or fizzy drinks.

Seasons—Acne often improves with natural sunlight and is worse in winter. The effect of artificial ultraviolet light is unpredictable.

External factors—Oils, whether vegetable oils in the case of cooks in hot kitchens or mineral oils in engineering, can cause "oil folliculitis", leading to acne like lesions. Other acnegenic substances include coal tar, dicophane (DDT), cutting oils, and halogenated hydrocarbons (polychlorinated biphenols and related chemicals). Cosmetic acne is seen in adult women who have used cosmetics containing comedogenic oils over many years.

Iatrogenic—Corticosteroids, both topical and systemic, can cause increased keratinisation of the pilosebaceous duct. Androgens, gonadotrophins, and corticotrophin can induce acne in adolescence. Oral contraceptives of the combined type can induce acne, and antiepileptic drugs are reputed to cause acne.

Hormones—the cause of all the trouble	
Androgens	increase the size of sebaceous glands
	increase sebum secretion
Androgenic adrenocorticosteroids have the same effect	
Oestrogens	have the opposite effect

Types of acne

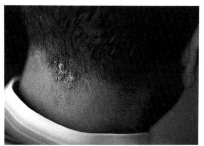

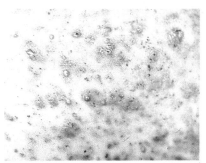

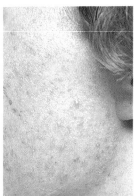

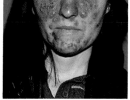

Acne keloidalis.

Acne vulgaris

Acne vulgaris, the common type of acne, occurs during puberty and affects the comedogenic areas of the face, back, and chest. There may be a familial tendency to acne. Acne vulgaris is slightly more common in boys, 30–40% of whom have acne between the ages of 18 and 19. In girls the peak incidence is between 16 and 18 years. Adult acne is a variant, affecting 1% of men and 5% of women aged 40. Acne keloidalis is a type of scarring acne seen on the neck in men.

Patients with acne often complain of excessive greasiness of the skin, with "blackheads", "pimples", or "plukes" developing. These may be associated with inflammatory papules and pustules developing into larger cysts and nodules. Resolving lesions leave inflammatory macules and scarring. Scars may be atrophic, sometimes with "ice pick" lesions or keloid formation. Keloids consist of hypertrophic scar tissue and occur predominantly on the neck, upper back, and shoulders and over the sternum.

Infantile acne—Localised acne lesions occur on the face in the first few months of life. They clear spontaneously but may last for some years. There is said to be an associated increased tendency to severe adolescent acne.

Acne conglobata—This is a severe form of acne, more common in boys and in tropical climates. It is extensive, affecting the trunk, face, and limbs. In "acne fulminans" there is associated systemic illness with malaise, fever, and joint pains. It appears to be associated with a hypersensitivity to *P. acnes*. Another variant is pyoderma faciale, which produces erythematous and necrotic lesions and occurs mainly in adult women.

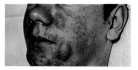

Acne conglobata.

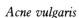

Acne fulminans.

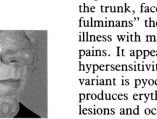

Pyoderma faciale.

Acne vulgaris
   affects comedogenic areas
   occurs mainly in puberty,
      in boys more than girls
   familial tendency

Infantile acne
   face only
   clears spontaneously

Severe acne
   acne conglobata
   pyoderma faciale
   Gram negative folliculitis

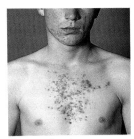

Acne vulgaris.

Occupational acne
   oils
   coal and tar
   chlorinated phenols
   DDT and weedkillers

Hormones
   combined type of oral
   contraceptives and
   androgenic hormones

Steroids
   systemic or topical

Gram negative folliculitis.

Gram negative folliculitis occurs with a proliferation of organisms such as klebsiella, proteus, pseudomonas, and *Escherichia coli*.

Occupational—Acne like lesions occur as a result of long term contact with oils or tar as mentioned above. This usually occurs as a result of lubricating, cutting, or crude oil soaking through clothing. In chloracne there are prominent comedones on the face and neck. It is caused by exposure to polychlortriphenyl and related compounds and also to weedkiller and dicophane.

Treatment of acne

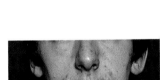

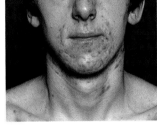

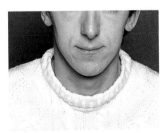

Before and after treatment with tetracycline.

In most adolescents acne clears spontaneously with minimal scarring. Reassurance and explanation along the following lines helps greatly:
   (1) The lesions can be expected to clear in time.
   (2) It is not infectious.
   (3) The less sufferers are self conscious and worry about their appearance the less other people will take any notice of their acne.

It helps to give a simple regimen to follow, enabling patients to take some positive steps to clear their skin and also an alternative to picking their spots.

I advise patients with acne to hold a hot wet flannel on the face (a much simpler alternative to the commercial "facial saunas"), followed by gentle rubbing in of a plain soap. Savlon solution, diluted 10 times with water, is an excellent alternative for controlling greasy skin.

There are many proprietary preparations, most of which act as keratolytics, dissolving the keratin plug of the comedone. They can also cause considerable dryness and scaling of the skin.

Benzoyl peroxide in concentrations of 1% to 10% comes as lotions, creams, gels, and washes. Resorcinol, sulphur, and salicylic acid preparations are also available.

Vitamin A acid as a cream or gel is helpful in some patients. A topical tretinoin gel has recently been introduced.

Ultraviolet light therapy is less effective than natural sunlight but is helpful for extensive acne.

Oral treatment—The mainstay of treatment is oxytetracycline, which should be given for a week at 1 g daily then 500 mg (250 mg twice daily) on an empty stomach. Minocycline or doxycycline are alternatives that can be taken with food. Perseverance with treatment is important, and it may take some months to produce an appreciable improvement. Erythromycin is an alternative to tetracycline, and co-trimoxazole can be used for Gram negative folliculitis. Tetracycline might theoretically interfere with the action of progesterone types of birth control pill and should not be given in pregnancy.

Topical antibiotics—Erythromycin, the tetracyclines, and clindamycin have been used topically. There is the risk of producing colonies of resistant organisms.

Acne and rosacea

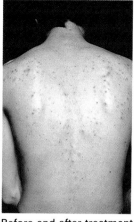

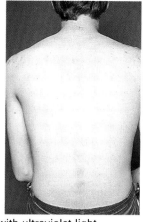

Before and after treatment with ultraviolet light.

Antiandrogens—Cyproterone acetate combined with ethinyloestradiol is effective in some women; it is also a contraceptive.

Synthetic retinoids—For severe cases resistant to other treatments these drugs, which can be prescribed only in hospital, are very effective and clear most cases in a few months. 13-*cis*-Retinoic acid (isotretinoin) is usually used for acne. They are teratogenic, so there must be no question of pregnancy, and can cause liver changes with raised serum lipid values. Regular blood tests are therefore essential. A three month course of treatment usually gives a long remission. Recently topical isotretinoin gel has been introduced.

Ultraviolet light is a helpful additional treatment in the winter months.

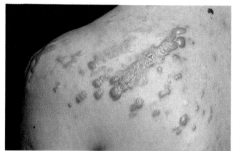

Keloid scars.

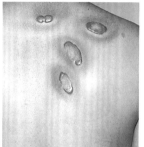

Keloid scars on dark skin.

Residual lesions, keloid scars, cysts, and persistent nodules can be treated by injection with triamcinolone or freezing with liquid nitrogen. For severe scarring dermabrasion can produce good cosmetic results. This is usually carried out in a plastic surgery unit.

Remember the following points

(1) Avoid topical steroids
(2) Persevere with one antibiotic not short courses of different types
(3) Do not prescribe a tetracycline for children and pregnant women
(4) Oxytetracycline must be taken on an empty stomach half an hour before meals

---

Treatment of acne

First line

(1) Encourage positive attitudes
(2) Avoid environmental and occupational factors
(3) Topical treatment
   Benzoyl peroxide
   Salicylic acid
(4) A tetracycline by mouth for several months

Second line

(1) Topical vitamin A acid
(2) Topical antibiotics
(3) Ultraviolet light
(4) Antiandrogens

Third line

Oral retinoids for 3–4 months (hospitals only)

Rosacea

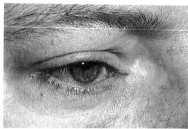

Blepharitis.

Rosacea is a persistent eruption occurring on the forehead and cheeks. It is more common in women than men.

There is erythema with prominent blood vessels. Pustules, papules, and oedema occur. Rhinophyma, with thickened erythematous skin of the nose and enlarged follicles, is a variant. Conjunctivitis and blepharitis may be associated. It is usually made worse by sunlight.

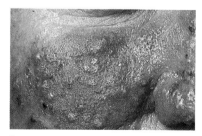

Rosacea.

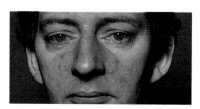

Rosacea.

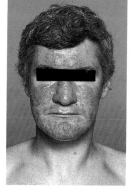

Rosacea.

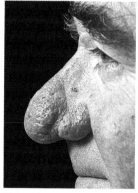

Rhinophyma.

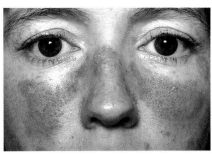

Lupus erythematosus.

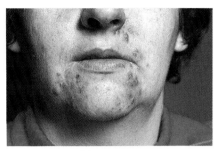

Perioral dermatitis.

Rosacea should be distinguished from:

Acne, in which there are blackheads, a wider distribution, and improvement with sunlight. Acne, however, may coexist with rosacea—hence the older term "acne rosacea".

Seborrhoeic eczema, in which there are no pustules and eczematous changes are present.

Lupus erythematosus, which shows light sensitivity, erythema, and scarring but no pustules.

Perioral dermatitis, which occurs in women with pustules and erythema around the mouth and on the chin. There is usually a premenstrual exacerbation. Treatment is with oral tetracyclines.

Treatment

The treatment of rosacea is with long term courses of oxytetracycline, which may need to be repeated. Topical treatment along the lines of that for acne is also helpful. Topical steroids should not be used as they have minimal effect and cause a severe rebound erythema, which is difficult to clear. Avoiding hot and spicy foods may help.

Recent reports indicate that synthetic retinoids are also effective.

Further reading

Cunliffe WJ, Cotterill JA. *The acnes: clinical features, pathogenesis and treatment.* St Louis: Mosby, 1989.
Plewig G, Kligman AM. *Acne and rosacea.* 2nd ed. Berlin: Springer Verlag, 1992.

11. BACTERIAL INFECTION

The process of infection involves the interaction of two organisms—host and invader. The clinical changes are a manifestation of the resulting "battle of the cells" as so clearly perceived by Metchnikoff 100 years ago. The lesions produced may have a well recognised appearance, such as impetigo or tinea cruris, but are often less specific.

Several features enable us to recognise that infection is a possible cause of the patient's condition.

Acute bacterial infections produce the classical characteristics of acute inflammation described by Celsus (see box).

Presentation

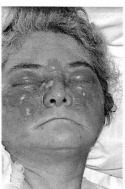 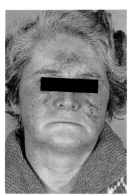

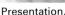

Presentation.   Two weeks later.

This woman had acute *erysipelas* due to haemolytic streptococcus, and all four features were present. She was, however, referred to the clinic with a diagnosis of acute allergy, which, from the appearance alone, was understandable. However, malaise and fever were also present and the lesions were warm. The condition responded well to antibiotic treatment. The point of entry in such cases may be a "spot" on the face or a small erosion near the nose, mouth, or ears. Erysipelas of the leg or foot may follow a small fissure between the toes.

Erysipelas is the local manifestation of a streptococcal infection, but this organism in the throat can result in the widespread rash of scarlet fever, which is rarely seen these days, or erythema multiforme, which is more common. An acute generalised vasculitis can also be associated with a streptococcal infection.

(1) In any patient with a localised area of acute erythema, swelling, and raised temperature consider infection

(2) Remember that a *generalised* erythematous rash may be the manifestation of a *localised* infection. Scarlet fever arises from streptococcal throat infection, and herpes simplex of the lip may be associated with erythema multiforme

(3) The common pathogens are also commensals—recent studies showed that 60% of individuals are nasal carriers of *Staphylococcus aureus* intermittently and 10% carry *Streptococcus pyogenes* in the throat

More chronic forms of bacterial infection include *impetigo, folliculitis, carbuncles*, and *ecthyma*. These conditions are due to streptococci and particularly to staphylococci, which are adept at colonising the skin, commonly in those with atopic eczema. Bacterial infection occurs in eczematous lesions and may itself cause an exacerbation of eczema.

Impetigo is a superficial infection of the skin, with transient blisters in the non-bullous form that then form crusts. Both staphylococci and streptococci are responsible. The bullous form is due to staphylococci.

Folliculitis, with infection and inflammatory changes in the upper follicle, is common. Deeper forms occur in the scalp (follicular impetigo) or the beard area (sycosis barbae). Abscess formation in the hair follicles results in furuncles or boils; several may coalesce to form a carbuncle.

Ecthyma, which is most common on the leg, is due to bacterial infection causing a necrotic lesion with a superficial crust and surrounding inflammation. Both streptococci and staphylococci are responsible.

Mycobacterial disease

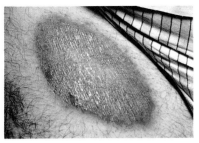

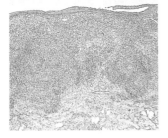

Lupus vulgaris.

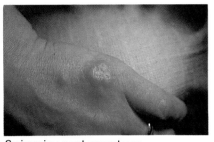

Swimming pool granuloma.

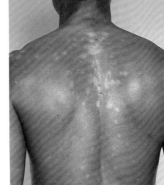

Tuberculoid leprosy.

The clinical presentation of mycobacterial disease depends on the immune response of the host—hence the difference between disseminated miliary tuberculosis and lupus vulgaris or, for example, tuberculoid and lepromatous leprosy.

These infections are rarely seen in the West so only the most common types—lupus vulgaris and "atypical mycobacterial infection" are described.

Lupus vulgaris is a very slowly growing indolent condition of the skin. The lesion shown had been present for 20 years and may have been acquired from the cattle with which the man worked. The characteristic giant cell granuloma can be clearly seen.

Atypical mycobacterial infections—Although infection with *Mycobacterium tuberculosis* is now rare in Britain, other types of mycobacterial skin infection occur. The most common is "fishtank" or "swimming pool" granuloma, aquired from tropical fish tackle or swimming pools, respectively, and caused by *Mycobacterium marinum*. Nodular lesions develop slowly with ulceration but there is no regional lymph node enlargement. *Mycobacterium kansasii* infection is rare and *Mycobacterium ulcerans* confined to the tropics.

Erythema of the face

Acute

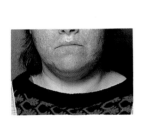

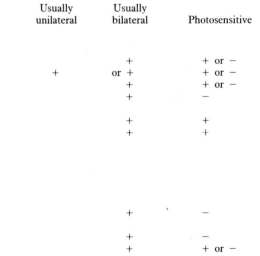

	Usually unilateral	Usually bilateral	Photosensitive
(1) Allergic reactions			
Cosmetics (*left*)		+	+ or −
Plants	+	or +	+ or −
Drugs		+	+ or −
(2) Urticaria		+	−
Reactions to light			
(3) Photodermatitis (*right*)		+	+
Solar urticaria		+	+
(4) Infection			
Erysipelas (*left*)		+	−
Fifth disease ("slapped cheek")		+	−
(5) Rosacea (*right*)		+	+ or −
(6) Lupus erythematosus			
Systemic (*left*)		+	+
Discoid (*right*)	+	or +	+
(7) Seborrhoeic dermatitis (*left*)		+	−
(8) Acne		+	+
(9) Perioral dermatitis (*right*)		+	−

Chronic-recurrent

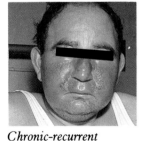

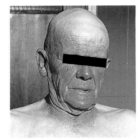

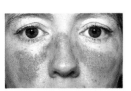

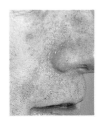

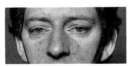

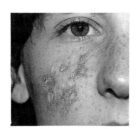

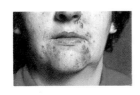

Common patterns of cutaneous bacterial infection

	Infected eczema	*Impetigo (non-bullous)*	*Impetigo (bullous)*
Appearance	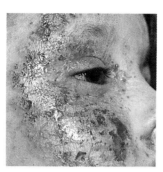	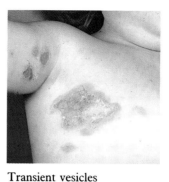	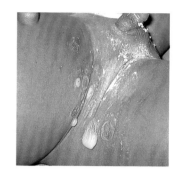
	Exudate Crusts Inflammation	Transient vesicles Exuding lesions with yellow crusts Erythema Affects mainly face and limbs, commonly in children	Erythema and bullae which rupture to leave superficial crusts May be central clearing Affects face, buttocks, and limbs in children and adults
Cause	Persistent scratching Topical steroids	Local reaction between invading organisms and neutrophils, resulting in superficial epidermal split in bullous lesion	
Organism	*Staphylococcus aureus* *Streptococcus pyogenes*	*Staphylococcus aureus* *Streptococcus pyogenes* in some outbreaks	*Staphylococcus aureus*
Treatment	(1) Weaker topical steroids (for the eczema) with topical antibiotics (2) Systemic antibiotics if necessary (3) Soaks with potassium permanganate (4) 1% eosin or gentian violet to paint erosions	Topical antibiotics Systemic antibiotics directed against both streptococcal and staphylococcal infection	Topical and systemic antibiotics
Notes	• Avoid prolonged use of topical antibiotics • Return to using weaker steroid when infection has healed • Even without clinical evidence of infection most lesions of atopic eczema are colonised by *Staphylococcus aureus*	• Staphylococcal infection can cause widespread superficial shedding of the epidermis—"scalded skin syndrome" (Lyell's disease) • It is wise to send a specimen for bacteriology: nephritogenic strains of streptococcus in impetigo remain an important cause for glomerulonephritis, although this is a rare condition.	

Boils (and furuncles) and carbuncles	Folliculitis	Ecthyma	Erysipelas
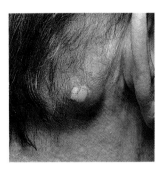	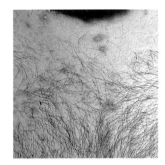	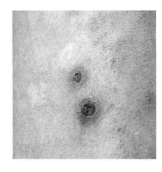	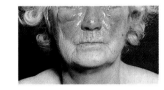
Inflammatory nodule affecting the hair follicles develops into a pustule Tender induration with considerable inflammation, followed by necrosis Heals with scarring More common in adolescents in winter Several boils may coalesce to form a carbuncle	Various forms: (1) *Scalp* *Children*—"Follicular impetigo" *Adults*— (*a*) Folliculitis cheloidalis Back of neck (*b*) Acne necrotica Forehead/hairline (2) *Face*—"Sycosis barbae" in men with seborrhoea (greasy skin) (3) *Legs*—Chronic folliculitis	Small bullae may be present initially An adherent crust is followed by a purulent ulcerated lesion with surrounding erythema and induration, which slowly heals Usually on legs	Well defined areas of erythema—very tender, not oedematous Vesicles may form Common sites—abdominal wall in infants; in adults the lower leg and face An area of broken skin, forming a portal of entry, may be found
Possible anaemia and fatigue Mechanical damage from clothing	(1) Underlying disease—e.g. diabetes (2) Infection may be precipitated by mechanical injury, tar pastes, and occlusive dressings	Minor injuries More common in debilitated individuals	Lymphoedema and severe inflammation due to bacterial toxins
Staphylococcus aureus, usually of same strain as in nose and perineum	*Staphylococcus aureus* *Propionibacterium acnes* *Pityrosporum* spp. *Pseudomonas* spp. and other Gram negative organisms	Both streptococcus and staphylococcus	*Streptococcus pyrogenes* (group A, but may be B, C, or G) *Staphylococcus aureus* *Klebsiella pneumoniae* *Haemophilus influenzae*
(1) Antibiotic (penicillinase resistant) systemically (2) Cleaning of skin with weak chlorhexedine solution or a similar preparation	Topical and long term systemic antibiotics—e.g. oxytetracycline Topical antifungal for pityrosporum infection	Improve nutrition Use antibiotic effective against both staphylococcus and streptococcus	Penicillin or erythromycin

- Nasal and perineal swabs should be taken to identify carriers
- Remember unusual causes—a bricklayer presented with a boil on the arm with necrosis due to anthrax (malignant pustule) acquired from the packing straw used for the bricks

- Gram negative folliculitis occurs on the face—a complication of long term treatment for acne
- A persistent, painful type of necrotic folliculitis occurs in those who wear hats, caps, or helmets for long periods

- Check for debilitating diseases, reticuloses, diabetes

- Cellulitis affects the deeper tissues and has more diverse causes, being essentially inflammation of the connective tissue
- Streptococcus, staphylococcus, haemophilus, and other organisms may be found
- Beware of erysipelas of the face—the venous drainage is deep to the cavernous sinus. A young resident physician decided to "tough out" her erysipelas on the cheek and refused treatment. Severe fever, facial oedema, and malaise associated with cavernous sinus phlebitis followed

Further reading
Canizares O, Harman RM. *Clinical tropical dermatology*. 2nd ed. Oxford: Blackwell Scientific, 1992.
Noble WC. *The skin: microflora and microbial skin disease*. Cambridge: Cambridge University Press, 1993.

12. VIRAL INFECTIONS

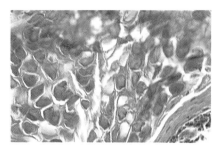

Molluscum inclusion bodies (a pox virus).

Like the pyogenic bacteria, viruses produce local lesions and may cause a widespread reaction to the infection. The clinical manifestations of common viral infections of the skin are well known and easily recognised.

Local infective lesions are caused by DNA viruses which can be isolated from the lesions themselves and include the herpes and pox groups.

In patients with AIDS florid and widespread viral infections of the skin occur.

Herpes

Herpes simplex

The herpes simplex virus consists of two antigenic types. Type I is associated with lesions on the face and fingers and sometimes genital lesions. Type II is associated almost entirely with genital infections.

Primary herpes simplex (type I) infection usually occurs in or around the mouth, with variable involvement of the face. Although there is usually a small area of inflammation with irritation forming a vesicle, there may be considerable inflammation and necrosis with malaise, probably depending on the degree of protection from maternal antibodies. Subsequent recurrent chronic infection of the lips may be due to virus remaining in the sensory nerve ganglia.

Type II infection affects the genitalia, vagina, and cervix and may predispose to cervical dysplasia

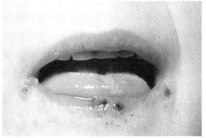

Herpes of lips.

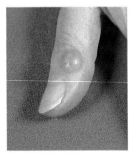 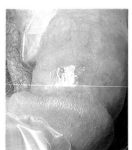

Inoculation herpes.   Genital herpes.

Herpes simplex—significant points

- The initial vesicular stage may not be seen in genital lesions, which present as painful ulcers or erosions
- There is usually a history of preceding itching and tenderness
- Scrapings from the base of the ulcer can be stained for viral inclusion bodies (Tzanck smears). The virus can often be cultured from vesicle fluid. Viral antigen can be shown by immunofluorescence
- Genital herpes in a pregnant woman carries a great risk of ophthalmic infection of the infant. Caesarean section may be indicated
- "Eczema herpeticum" or "Kaposi's varicelliform eruption" are terms applied to life-threatening systemic infection with herpes virus in patients with atopic eczema and some other skin conditions. Treatment is with parenteral acyclovir. It can also be caused by vaccinia and coxsackie viruses

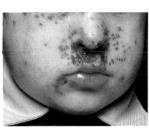 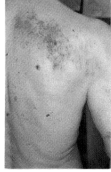

Eczema herpeticum   Herpes zoster.

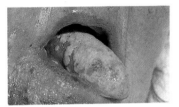

Mandibular zoster.

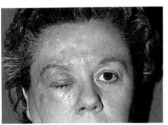

Ophthalmic zoster.

Pox viruses

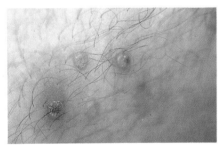

Molluscum contagiosum.

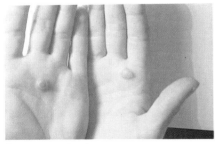

Cowpox, early stage.

Herpes zoster

Herpes zoster, due to herpesvirus varicella, which also causes chickenpox (due to a herpes virus, not a pox virus), develops without a definable incubation period. There is, however, often pain, fever, and malaise before erythematous papules develop in the area of the affected dermatome—most commonly in the thoracic area. Vesicles develop over several days, leaving dried crusts as they resolve. Secondary infection is common. The subsequent neuralgia, particularly in elderly people, is well known.

Remember that infection from both skin lesions and nasopharyngeal secretions can cause chickenpox.

Treatment

The usual troublesome, localised lesions of herpes simplex have been treated with topical zinc sulphate, iodoxuridine, ice cubes, and photoactivation of eosin. Topical acyclovir—a drug that inhibits herpes virus DNA polymerase—is effective and should be used as soon as the patient is aware of symptoms.

Severe, recurrent, herpes simplex or herpes zoster can be treated with acyclovir by mouth or injection, given as early in the course of the illness as possible.

Secondary infection may require antiseptic soaks, such as 1/1000 potassium permanganate, or topical or systemic antibiotics.

Steroids (prednisolone 40–60 mg/day) given during the acute stage of herpes zoster diminish pain and postherpetic neuralgia.

Rest and analgesics are recommended treatment for extensive herpes simplex or herpes zoster infections.

> **Steroids should not be given to immunodeficient patients, in whom they may cause disseminated infection**

The pox viruses are also large DNA viruses, particularly infecting the epidermis.

Variola (smallpox), once the cause of high mortality, has been officially eliminated by vaccination with modified vaccinia virus—the culmination of Jenner's pioneer work.

Molluscum contagiosum

The commonest "pox" seen these days is molluscum contagiosum—a worry to mothers of affected infants, who are not themselves unduly concerned. Despite its name it is not very contagious, except in overcrowded conditions in tropical countries. In temperate climates it often affects only one or two children in a household.

In adults florid molluscum contagiosum may be an indication of underlying immunodeficiency, as in AIDS patients.

Clinical features—The white, umbilicated papules of molluscum contagiosum are characteristic. Large solitary lesions may cause confusion and so can secondarily infected, excoriated lesions. Remember that these can itch, particularly in patients with atopy. There may be widespread lesions in patients with AIDS and which are said to be more common in sarcoidosis and atopy.

Diagnosis is not difficult. Sometimes there is confusion with viral warts and, in a solitary lesion, a benign tumour of the skin.

Treatment—Most treatments are painful and should not be inflicted on a child with a benign self limiting condition. An antibiotic-hydrocortisone ointment can be used for excoriated lesions. Treatment with liquid nitrogen is probably the simplest treatment. Other methods include superficial curettage and carefully rotating a sharpened orange stick moistened with phenol in the centre of each lesion.

Other pox infections

The other pox infections are of incidental interest.

Cowpox only sporadically infects cows from its natural reservoir, probably small mammals, and may affect humans. Papules on the hands enlarge and develop necrosis and crusting.

Viral infections

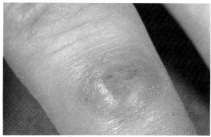

Milkers' nodule

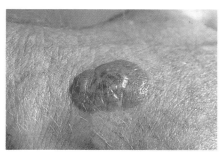

Orf.

Milkers' nodules are due to a virus that causes superficial ulcers in cows' udders and calves' mouths. In humans papules form on the hands and develop into grey nodules with a necrotic centre, surrounding inflammation, and lymphangeitis. A more generalised papular eruption can occur.

Orf is easily diagnosed by country doctors, sheep farmers, and veterinarians but may be overinvestigated by those less familiar with rural dermatology. It is seen mainly in early spring as a result of contact with lambs. A single papule or group of lesions develops on the fingers or hands with purple papules developing into a bulla. This ruptures to leave an annular lesion 1–3 cm in diameter with a necrotic centre. There is surrounding inflammation. The incubation period is a few days and the lesions last 2–3 weeks with spontaneous healing. Associated erythema multiforme and widespread rashes are occasionally seen.

Monkey pox, *reindeer pox*, and *musk ox pox* are of interest to those treating zookeepers and travellers.

Wart viruses

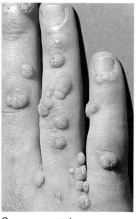

Common warts.

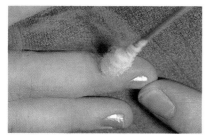

Treatment with liquid nitrogen.

The true worth of the papilloma virus, which causes warts, as an object of serious study has only recently been recognised. The wart is, after all, one of the few tumours in which a virus can be seen to proliferate in the cell nucleus. The different kinds of wart are caused by a very wide range of papilloma virus, currently divided into over 80 major types. These are classified into three categories—*cutaneous*, *mucocutaneous* and *epidermodysplasia verruciformis*. The following aspects should be remembered:

● Genital warts (due to human papilloma virus) very rarely undergo malignant change but the associated infection of the cervix frequently leads to dysplasia or malignant changes. Cervical smears must be taken.

● Very extensive proliferation of warts occurs in patients receiving immunosuppressive therapy, such as renal transplant recipients, and in patients with AIDS.

● Epidermodysplasia verruciformis, an unusual widespread eruption of erythematous warty plaques, can develop into carcinoma.

Treatment

Most warts occur in childen and resolve spontaneously without treatment or with very simple measures. These include paints or lotions containing salicylic and lactic acids and formalin in various proportions, which should be applied daily. Salicylic acid (40%) plasters are useful for plantar warts; they are cut to shape and held in place with sticking plaster for two or three days. Glutaraldehyde solution is also used.

For warts that get in the way, are painful, or are disfiguring more drastic measures can be used:

(1) *Cold*—Carbon dioxide snow is readily produced from a cylinder and can be mixed with acetone to form a slush. This is applied with a cotton wool swab. Liquid nitrogen is colder and more effective but has to be stored in special containers and replaced frequently. It can be applied with cotton wool or discharged from a special spray apparatus. Freezing is continued until there is a rim of frozen tissue around the wart but not for more than 30 seconds. Subsequent blistering may occur. Scarring is unusual.

(2) *Heat*—Cautery causes more scarring and requires local anaesthesia. The diathermy loop is effective for perianal warts.

(3) *Curettage and cautery* together are effective but leave scars and the warts may recur.

(4) *Podophyllin*, 15–25% in tincture of benzoin compound or alcoholic solution, is effective for genital warts when applied each week. It is, however, toxic when ingested or absorbed and must never be used in pregnancy.

Other treatments include radiotherapy, fluorouracil, and bleomycin injections. Hypnosis has been effectively used, and fear of painful treatment has caused warts to fall off.

Virus diseases with rashes

Measles
Rubella
Infectious mononucleosis
Erythema infectiosum
Roseola infantum
Gianotti–Crosti syndrome
Hand, foot, and mouth disease
Primary HIV infection

Measles and rubella, which were once familiar to every doctor, are now much less common as a result of widespread inoculation. However, measles is probably the best known example of an exanthem (a fever characterised by a skin eruption. In an enanthem the mucous surfaces are affected.) Other common clinical patterns can then be compared with it. All exanthems, except fifth disease (erythema infectiosum), are due to RNA viruses.

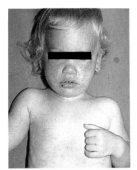

Measles.

Measles

Age—Measles affects children, usually those aged over 5.

Incubation lasts seven to 14 days.

Prodromal symptoms include fever, malaise, upper respiratory symptoms; conjunctivitis; and photophobia.

Initial rash—Early on Koplik's spots (white spots with surrounding erythema) appear on the oral mucosa. After two days a macular rash appears on the face, trunk, and limbs. Look behind the ears for early lesions.

Development and resolution—The rash becomes papular, with coalescence. There may be haemorrhagic lesions and bullae which fade to leave brown patches.

Complications are encephalitis, otitis media, and bronchopneumonia.

Diagnosis—Specific antibodies may be detected; they are at their maximum at two to four weeks.

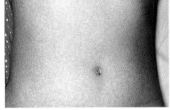

Rubella.

Rubella

Age—Rubella affects children and young adults.

Incubation lasts 14–21 days.

Prodromal symptoms—There are none in young children. Otherwise fever, malaise, and upper respiratory symptoms occur.

Initial rash—Initially some patients develop erythema of the soft palate and lymphadenopathy. Later pink macules appear on the face, spreading to trunk and limbs over one to two days.

Development and resolution—The rash then clears over the next two days, and sometimes no rash develops at all.

Complications—The main complication is congenital defects in babies of women infected during pregnancy. The risk is greatest in the first month.

Diagnosis—The diagnosis is made from the clinical signs above. Serum should be taken for measuring antibodies and the test repeated at seven to 10 days.

Prophylaxis—Active immunisation is now routinely available for all schoolgirls.

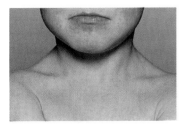

Erythema infectiosum.

Erythema infectiosum (fifth disease)

Age group—Erythema infectiosum affects children aged 2–10 years, mainly girls.

Incubation lasts five to 20 days.

Prodromal symptoms—There are usually none, but there may be a slight fever with initial rash.

Initial rash—The initial rash is a hot, erythematous eruption on the cheeks—hence the "slapped cheek syndrome." Over two to four days a maculopapular eruption develops on the arms, legs, and trunk.

Development and resolution—The rash extends to affect hands, feet, and mucous membranes, then fades over one to two weeks.

Diagnosis is made by finding a specific IgM antibody to parvovirus B19.

Complications—There are no reported dermatological complications but haematological disorders, arthropathy, and fetal abnormalities may be associated.

Viral infections

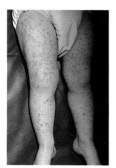

Gianotti–Crosti syndrome.

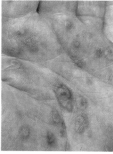

Hand, foot, and mouth disease.

Roseola infantum

Age group—Roseola infantum affects infants aged under 2.

Incubation lasts 10–15 days.

Prodromal symptoms—There is fever for a few days.

Initial rash—A rose pink maculopapular eruption appears on the neck and trunk.

Development and resolution—The rash may affect the face and limbs before clearing over one to two days.

Diagnosis—The condition is diagnosed from its clinical features.

Complications include febrile convulsions.

Gianotti-Crosti syndrome

Age group—The Gianotti-Crosti syndrome affects children, usually those aged under 14.

Incubation period is unknown.

Prodromal symptoms—Lymphadenopathy and malaise accompany the eruption.

Initial rash—Red papules rapidly develop on the face, neck, limbs, buttocks, palms, and soles.

Development and resolution—Over two to three weeks the lesions become purpuric then slowly fade.

Diagnosis—The syndrome may be due to a number of virus infections. Check for hepatitis B antigen.

Complications—Lymphadenopathy and hepatomegaly always occur and may persist for many months.

Hand, foot, and mouth disease

Age—Hand, foot, and mouth disease (Coxsackie virus A) affects both children and adults.

Incubation period is unknown.

Prodromal symptoms—Fever, headache, and malaise may accompany the rash.

Initial rash—Initially there may be intense erythema surrounding yellow-grey vesicles; ulceration then occurs. This pattern is more common in adults. Alternatively, there may be grey vesicles, 1–5 mm diameter, with surrounding erythema on the palms and soles. These occur mainly in children, in whom a more generalised eruption may develop.

Development and resolution—Over three to five days the rash fades.

Diagnosis—Coxsackie A (usually A16) virus is isolated from lesions and stools. A specific antibody may be found in the serum.

Complications are rare but include widespread vesicular rashes and erythema multiforme.

Other infections

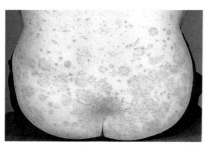

Secondary syphilis.

Infectious mononucleosis—As well as the erythematous lesions on the palate a maculopapular rash affecting the face and limbs can occur.

Cat scratch disease—A crusted nodule at the site of the scratch is associated with development of regional lymphadenopathy one or two months later. A maculopapular eruption on the face and limbs or erythema multiforme may occur.

Psittacosis and ornithosis may be associated with a rash.

Rickettsial infections, including typhus, Rocky Mountain spotted fever, and Rickettsial pox are all associated with rashes.

Syphilis—Although not a viral infection, the transient roseolar rash of secondary syphilis is followed by a papulosquamous eruption, which affects the trunk, limbs, and mucous membranes. The palms and soles may be affected. The diagnosis should always be considered in any rash that does not fit a recognised pattern.

Further reading

Joklik WK. *Virology*. 3rd ed. Norwalk: Appleton and Lange, 1988.

Mandell GL, Douglas RG, Bennett JF. *Principles and practice of infectious diseases*. 3rd ed. New York: Churchill Livingstone, 1990.

Timbury MC. *Notes on medical virology*. 9th ed. Edinburgh: Churchill Livingstone, 1991.

White DO, Fenner FJ. *Medical virology*. 4th ed. New York: Academic Press, 1994.

13. HIV and AIDS

Since AIDS was first described in 1981 over 400 000 cases have been reported to the World Health Organisation, but the total is probably much larger. In Europe the figure is over 60 000, of which 5000 are from the United Kingdom. The number of people infected with HIV is much larger. It is generally accepted that this retrovirus is the causative agent of AIDS, but its origins remain unknown.

Skin lesions occur in patients with AIDS:
- As a manifestation of the primary HIV infection.
- As a consequence of immunosuppression (AIDS).

Between these two events there is a latent period that can last from a few months to several years. Lymphadenopathy may occur without other signs of the disease.

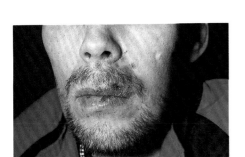
Seborrhoeic dermatitis.

Acute HIV infection (seroconversion illness) is associated with clinical changes in about a half of cases. Fever, malaise, headache, lymphadenopathy, and gastrointestinal upset occur. Sometimes there is an effect on the central nervous system. Soon after the onset of these effects a transient maculopapular eruption occurs, with erythema and erosion of the palate in some patients. At this time HIV can be isolated from circulating lymphocytes and HIV antibody testing may still give negative results, although an antigenaemia soon develops. For this reason it may be important to retest suspected cases 6–8 weeks later. Counselling should take place when testing is carried out.

Skin manifestations of AIDS and late stage HIV disease are many and variable. The main features are that the common inflammatory skin diseases are more florid, infections are frequent and severe, and opportunistic infections occur. In addition Kaposi's sarcoma occurs in 34% of homosexual men and in 5% of other cases.

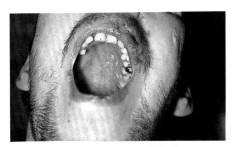
Herpes zoster with oral candidiasis.

Seborrhoeic eczema is common and may be the only evidence of HIV infection initially. It is more extensive and inflamed than usual. The role of *Pityrosporum* organisms is indicated by the response to imidazole antifungal drugs.

Psoriasis is more widespread, severe, and resistant to treatment in patients with late HIV disease. The use of ultraviolet light may lead to an increased risk of Kaposi's sarcoma.

Any type of opportunistic infection is more likely in patients with AIDS and will generally be more severe.

An itching, *inflammatory folliculitis* occurs in many cases. The cause is unknown, but it is possible that *Demodex* spp. play a part.

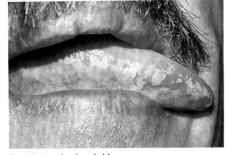
Oral hairy leukoplakia.

Herpes zoster virus infection is common, with florid lesions and systemic spread. Often two dermatomes are affected. *Herpes simplex virus* produces widespread and sometimes persistent ulcerating lesions.

61

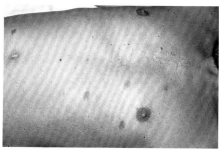

Kaposi's sarcoma.

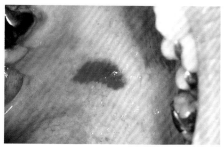

Kaposi's sarcoma of the hard palate.

Perianal warts can proliferate and *cervical intraepithelial neoplasia* occurs. *Molluscum contagiosum* is often widespread, particularly on the face.

Fungal infections may be widespread and with increased inflammation and hyperkeratosis. *Candidiasis*, often with associated bacterial infection, is very common, particularly at the corners of the mouth, on the palate, and in the pharynx.

Cryptococcus neoformans and *Histoplasma capsulatum* are occasional opportunistic pathogens and can produce inflammatory, papular, and necrotic lesions.

Mycobacteria may cause both cutaneous and systemic lesions.

Oral hairy leukoplakia may occur in 30–50% of patients with AIDS.

Kaposi's sarcoma presents with polychromic plaques and nodules, varying from red and purple to brown. They are common on the palate and nose, often found on the trunk, but can be disseminated or produce lesions in the classical site—the ankle.

AIDS may thus present with a wide variety of skin conditions, commonly with several present at the same time. Any unusually florid skin condition that is resistant to treatment should raise the suspicion that HIV infection may be present.

Further reading

Adler MW. *ABC of AIDS*. 4th ed. London: BMJ Publishing Group, 1997.
Penneys NS. *Skin manifestations of AIDS*. 2nd ed. St Louis: Mosby, 1995.

14. FUNGAL AND YEAST INFECTIONS

Fungal infections

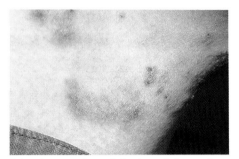

Tricophyton rubrum infection of the neck.

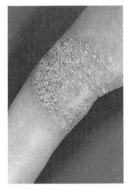

Animal ringworm.

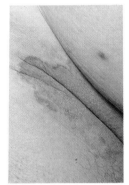

Tinea cruris.

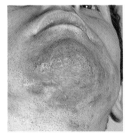

T. mentagrophytes.

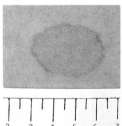

M. canis.

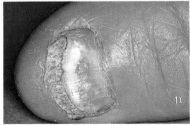

Fungal infection of nail.

Fungal infections are commonly known as "ringworm"—a misnomer since most infections cause a scaling macule, not a ring, and the worm exists only in the imagination. It is true, however, that a superficial fungal infection can have a raised edge, and annular forms occur.

Fungi consist of thread-like hyphae—which form tangled masses, or mycelia, in the common moulds. In "dermatophyte" fungal infection of the skin, hair, and nails these hyphae invade keratin and are seen on microscopic examination of keratin from infected tissues. Vegetative spores (conidia) develop in culture, and their distinctive shape helps to differentiate one species from another. Skin scrapings or clippings from infected nails can be easily taken and should always be sent to the laboratory for mycological examination and culture in any patient suspected of having a fungal infection.

Systemic, or deep, fungal infection is due to those species that invade other tissues. When the immune response is impaired superficial infections may invade the deeper tissues.

Yeasts are budding unicellular organisms that do not normally produce hyphae. The commonest infective species in humans is *Candida albicans*.

Why should one suspect a lesion to be due to a fungus?

Clinical presentation

Fungal infections usually itch. Those due to zoophilic (animal) fungi produce a more intense inflammatory response with deeper indurated lesions than those due to anthropophilic (human) species. In those lesions with a raised scaling margin that extends outwards the fungal hyphae are invading the keratin layer in this area. The central area is relatively resistant to colonisation. Such lesions occur mainly on the trunk.

Children below the age of puberty rarely develop anthropophilic (human) fungal infection. In the countryside cattle ringworm (zoophilic) infects children in the autumn when the cows are brought into winter quarters. Pet mice can also be a source of infection.

Adults—From adolescence onwards infection of the feet, not only in athletes, occurs. Tinea cruris in the groin is seen mainly in men.

Infection from cattle occurs in adults who have not had previous exposure, sometimes in unusual ways. A man who lived in an industrial area housing estate developed a curious indurated lesion on his chin from which *Trichophyton mentagrophytes* was isolated—transmitted by bites from midges who had been biting cows on a farm some miles away.

Infection from dogs and cats with a zoophilic fungus (*Microsporum canis*) to which humans have little immunity can occur at any age. A colleague's daughter returned from a skiing holiday with intensely itchy "eczema," which refused to clear. A stray kitten, mewing outside in the dark, had been taken indoors, warmed in their sleeping bags, and infected the whole party with *M. canis*.

Nail infections occur mainly in adults, usually in their toenails, especially when traumatised—for example, the big toes of footballers. The nails become thickened and yellow and crumble, usually asymmetrically. The changes occur *distally* and move back to the nailfold. In psoriasis of the nail the changes occur *proximally* and tend to be symmetrical and are associated with pitting and other evidence of psoriasis elsewhere.

Fungal and yeast infections

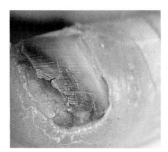

Chronic paronychia.

Chronic paronychia occurs in the fingers of individuals whose work demands repeated wetting of the hands: housewives, barmen, dentists, nurses, and mushroom growers, for example. Other predisposing factors include diabetes, poor peripheral circulation, and removal of the cuticle. There is erythema and swelling of the nail fold, often on one side with brownish discoloration of the nail. Pus may be exuded. The cause is *Candida albicans* (a yeast) together with secondary bacterial infection.

Pushing back the cuticles should be avoided. It is commonly a long term condition, lasting for years. The hands should be kept as dry as possible, nystatin cream applied regularly, and, if necessary a course of erythromycin prescribed.

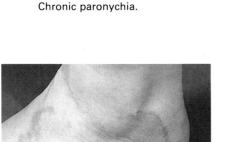

Tinea pedis.

Feet—It is not only athletes and the unhygienic who suffer from athletes' foot but increased sweating does predispose to infection. The hands may be affected, often through scratching the feet; hence the "right hand, left foot" syndrome in the right handed individual. The itching, macerated skin beneath the toes is familiar, but when a dry, scaling rash extends across the sole and dorsal surface of one foot the diagnosis may be missed. The condition needs to be differentiated from psoriasis and eczema.

Hands—Fungal infections often produce a dry, hot, rash on one palm. There may be well defined lesions with a scaling edge.

Trunk—Tinea corporis presents with erythema and itching and a well defined scaling edge. The infection may spread to the adjacent skin on the thighs and abdomen. Intense erythema and satellite lesions suggest a candida infection. In the axillae erythrasma due to *Corynebacterium minutissimum* is more likely. It does not respond to antifungal treatment but clears with tetracycline by mouth.

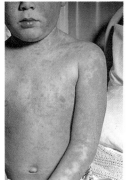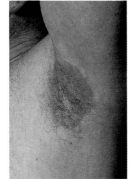

Tinea corporis.   Erythrasma.

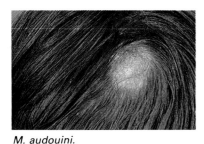

M. audouini.

Scalp and face—The classic scalp ringworm of children due to *Microsporum audouini* is rare. Favus, a scarring type of alopecia, caused by *Trichophyton schoenleini*, and "black dot" ringworm, also from a trichophyton, are now seen only in children who have acquired the infection abroad. In all cases there is itching, hair loss, and some degree of inflammation. *M. canis* from dogs and cats can affect the scalp.

Kerion—an inflamed, boggy, pustular lesion, is due to cattle ringworm and is fairly common in rural areas. It is often seen in children in the autumn when the cows are brought inside for the winter.

"*Tinea incognito*" is the term used for unrecognised fungal infection in patients treated with steroids (topical or systemic). The normal response to infection (leading to erythema, scaling, a raised margin, and itching) is diminished, particularly with local steroid creams or ointments. The infecting organism flourishes, however, because of the host's impaired immune response—shown by the enlarging, persistent skin lesions. The groins, hands, and face are sites where this is most likely to occur.

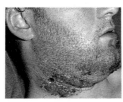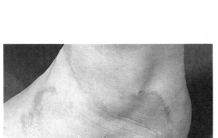

Tinea incognito.   Actinomycosis.

Deep fungal infection

Fungal infection of the deeper tissues is rare in the United Kingdom but is of course a feature of AIDS. The species that colonise the deep tissue, as in histoplasmosis, actinomycosis, and cryptococcosis, can also cause skin lesions. In any patient with chronic indurated inflammatory lesions the possibility of deep fungal infection should be considered.

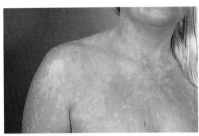

Tinea versicolor.

Tinea versicolor affects the trunk, usually of fair skinned individuals exposed to the sun. It affects mainly the upper back, chest, and arms. Well defined macular lesions with fine scales develop which tend to be white in suntanned areas and brown on pale skin (hence "versicolor"—variable colour). It may be confused with seborrhoeic dermatitis, pityriasis rosea, and vitiligo.

In skin scrapings the causative organism, *Pityrosporum* spp.—normally found in hair follicles—can be readily seen.

Yeast infections

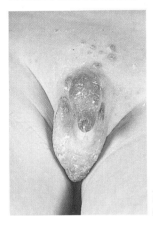

Candida albicans.

Candida infection may occur in the flexures of infants and elderly or immobilised patients, especially below the breasts and folds of abdominal skin. It needs to be differentiated from (*a*) psoriasis, which does not itch; (*b*) seborrhoeic dermatitis, the usual cause of a flexural rash in infants; and (*c*) contact dermatitis and discoid eczema, which do not have the scaling margin. It is symmetrical.

Yeasts, including *Candida albicans*, may be found in the mouth and vagina of healthy individuals. Clinical lesions may be produced by local trauma predisposing factors including: general debilitation, impaired immunity, diabetes mellitus, endocrine disorders, particularly Cushing's syndrome, and corticosteroid treatment. Florid mucocutaneous lesions can occur in which mycelial forms of *Candida albicans* are found.

Principles of diagnosis and treatment

(1) Consider a fungal infection in any patient where isolated, itching, dry, and scaling lesions occur without any apparent reason—for example, if there is no previous history of eczema. Lesions due to fungal infection are often asymmetrical.

(2) Skin scrapings should be sent to the laboratory from any suspicious lesion and are easy to take. The skin scales should be removed by scraping the edge of the lesion with a scalpel at right angles to the skin on to a piece of folded black paper. A strip of Sellotape applied to the lesion then stuck on a slide gives the laboratory more material for culture. Some laboratories supply mycology kits containing black paper, a slide with Sellotape, and suitable plastic containers. Clippings can be taken from the nails.

(3) Lesions to which steroids have been applied are often quite atypical because the normal inflammatory response is suppressed—tinea incognito. The patient often states that the treatment controls the itch but the contagion lingers on, becoming worse when the steroid is stopped. This may also occur in eczema being treated with steroids.

(4) Wood's light (ultraviolet light filtered through special glass) can be used to show microsporum infections, which produce a green-blue fluorescence.

Treatment

Topical treatment—The old fashioned treatment with Whitfield's ointment (benzoic acid ointment, compound) is quite effective, but has been superseded by the new imidazole preparations, such as clotrimazole and miconazole and also by terbinafine. The polyenes, nystatin and amphotericin B are also effective against yeast infection. For damp macerated skin dusting powders or painting with Castellani's paint (magenta paint) is helpful. Terbinafine, a fungicidal drug, is available as a cream and is very effective.

Systemic treatment—It is important to confirm the diagnosis from skin scrapings before starting treatment.

Terbinafine is a very effective fungicidal drug. It is taken in a dosage of 250 mg once daily for two to six weeks for skin infections and up to three months for finger nail infections or six months for toenail infections. It has not yet been approved for use in children. It should be administered with care in any form of liver disease or impaired renal function. Pregnancy and lactation are relative contraindications. There have been reports of headaches, joint pains, and liver dysfunction.

Imidazole preparations such as ketoconazole are effective in both dermatophyte fungi and yeast infections. Cases of liver damage have however been reported. Fluconazole is effective in yeast infections. Some drugs interact with azole drugs, the main ones being anticoagulants, oral hypoglycaemic drugs, phenytoin, and theophylline.

Griseofulvin should be taken for an adequate length of time, three to four months for the trunk and scalp, six to eight months for the finger nails, and at least a year for toenails where it is often ineffective. The dose is 500 mg daily for adults and 10 mg/kg for children, taken with food. Contraindications to griseofulvin are pregnancy, liver failure, and porphyria. It interacts with the coumarin anticoagulants and is made less effective by barbiturates.

Further reading

Conant NF. *Manual of clinical mycology.* 3rd ed. Philadelphia: Saunders, 1971.
Elewski BE. *Cutaneous fungal infections.* New York: Igaku-Shoin, 1992.
Evans EG, Richardson MD. *Medical mycology: a practical approach.* Oxford: Oxford University Press, 1989.

15. INSECT BITES AND INFESTATIONS

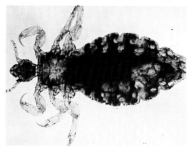

Body louse.

So, naturalists observe, a flea
Hath smaller fleas that on him prey;
And these have smaller fleas to bite 'em
And so proceed "Ad infinitum."

JONATHAN SWIFT

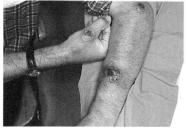

Leishmaniasis.

It is, of course, the internal parasites of biting insects that cause trouble for humans, rather than "smaller fleas" on their surface.

An ornithologist went bird watching in Guyana, where he sustained widespread "midge bites" on the arms. He was referred on account of nodules that developed a few weeks later, then enlarged and ulcerated. Other lesions occurred further up the arms with regional lymphadenopathy. A biopsy specimen showed histiocytic inflammatory changes, and *Leishmania braziliensis* was isolated from smears; the midges (*phlebotomus* or sand fly) had acquired the protozoon while feeding on local rodents and transferred it into the ornithologist's skin.

Serious disease from insect vectors is rare in residents of most Western countries but, as in the patient described above, must be considered in those returning from tropical and subtropical countries.

Most cases of bites from fleas, midges, and mosquitoes are readily recognised and cause few symptoms apart from discomfort. Occasionally an allergic reaction confuses the picture, particularly the large bullae that can occur from bites on the arms and legs. It may be difficult to persuade patients that their recurrent itching spots are simply due to flea bites and the suggestion may be angrily rejected.

Some diseases with skin lesions resulting from insect bites

Condition	Appearance	Organism	Vector
Cutaneous leishmaniasis	Chronic enlarging nodules with ulceration	Leishmania protozoon (L. braziliensis)	Sand fly
Oriental sore	Ulcerating nodules	Leishmania (L. tropica)	Sand fly
Kala-azar	Hypopigmented, erythematous, and nodular lesions	Leishmania (L. donovani)	Insect vectors
Onchocerciasis	Pruritic nodules	Filaria (Onchocerca volvulus)	Black fly (Simuliidae)
Typhus, human	Erythematous rash and systemic illness	Rickettsia (R. prowazekii)	Human louse
Typhus, murine		(R. mooseri)	Rat flea
Rocky Mountain spotted fever	Maculopapular rash and fever	Rickettsia (R. rickettsii)	Ticks
Rickettsial pox	Vesicular eruption like chickenpox	Rickettsia (R. akari)	House mouse, louse
Tick typhus	Necrotic lesions, maculopapular rash, and fever	Various rickettsias	Ticks
Scrub typhus	Fever, lymphadenopathy, maculopapular rash	Rickettsia (R. tsutsugamushi)	Mites
Relapsing fever	Widespread maculopapular lesions	Borrelia recurrentis	Lice, ticks
Lyme disease	May be annular	Borrelia burgdorferi	Ticks, black fly
Yellow fever and dengue	Flushing of face, scarlatiniform rash	Arbovirus	Aedes mosquito

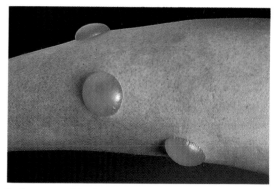

Bullae caused by insect bites.

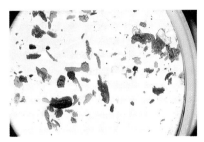

Parasitophobia specimens.

On the other hand, some patients are convinced that they have an infestation when they do not. Often they will bring small packets containing "insects". Examination shows these to be small screws of wool, pickings of keratin, thread, and so on. Sympathy and tact will win patients' confidence; derision and disbelief will merely send them elsewhere for a further medical opinion. Pimozide by mouth may help to dispel the delusion of parasitic infestation (delusional parasitosis).

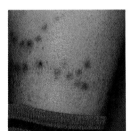

Bites on ankles.

Some useful points.

(1) Flea bites, including those from *Cheyletiella* mites in dogs and cats, occur in clusters, often in areas of close contact with clothing—for example, around the waist.

(2) Grain mites (*Pyemotes*) and harvest mites (*Trombiculidae*) can cause severe reactions.

(3) Tick, and possibly mosquito, bites can produce infection with *Borrelia burgdorferi*, causing arthropathy, fever, and a distinctive rash (erythema chronicum migrans)—Lyme disease. The condition responds rapidly to treatment with penicillin. Increasing numbers of cases are being reported in the United Kingdom.

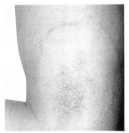

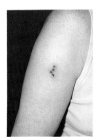

Erythema chronicum migrans.

Harvest mites.

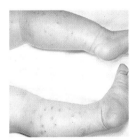

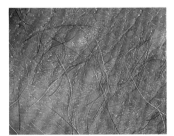

Papular urticaria.

Persistent papules in scabies.

Papular urticaria

Persistent pruritic (itching) papules in groups on the trunk and legs may be due to bites from fleas, bed bugs, or mites. A seasonal incidence suggests bites from outdoor insects, while recurrence of the papules in a particular house or room suggests infestations with fleas. The term is sometimes used for other causes of itchy skin.

Spider bites

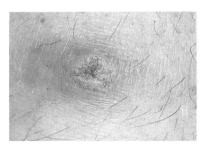

Spider bite (Nigeria).

In Europe spider bites rarely cause problems, but sometimes noxious species arrive in consignments of tropical fruit. The patient shown had been bitten by a spider the day before leaving Nigeria and developed a painful necrotic lesion.

Bites from the European tarantula are painful but otherwise harmless.

In tropical and subtropical countries venomous spiders inject neurotoxins that can be fatal. The "black widow" (*Latrodectus mactans*), "fiddleback" (*Loxosceles veclusa*), and *Atrax* species of Australia are better known examples. Scorpions cause severe local and systemic symptoms as a result of stings (not bites).

Infestations

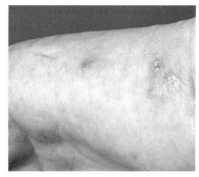

Burrows of scabies.

Scabies: points to note

- There may be very few burrows, though the patient has widespread itching

- The distribution of the infestation is characteristically the fingers, wrists, nipples, abdomen, genitalia, buttocks, and ankles. It does not occur above the neck

- Close personal contact is required for infestation to occur—e.g. within a family, through infants in playgroups, and through regular nursing of elderly patients

- Itching may persist even after all mites have been eliminated; itching papules on the scrotum and penis are particularly persistent

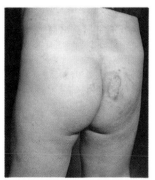

Larva migrans.

Scabies

The commonest infestation encountered is scabies, and it is easily missed or misdiagnosed. Scabies is due to a small mite, *Sarcoptes scabiei*. The female mite burrows into the stratum corneum to lay her eggs; the male dies after completing his role of fertilisation, and the developing eggs hatch into larvae within a few days. Intense itching occurs some two weeks later, during which time extensive colonisation may have occurred. The infestation is acquired only by close contact with infected people.

Diagnosis—Finding a burrow—the small (5–10 mm long) ridge, often S shaped—can be difficult as it is often obscured by excoriation from scratching. Without finding a burrow, however, the diagnosis remains uncertain. Isolation of an acarus with a needle or scalpel blade and its demonstration under the microscope convinces the most sceptical patient. Always ask whether there are others in the patient's household and if any of them are itching.

Treatment—10% Sulphur in yellow soft paraffin is traditional, effective, and safe. There are several more modern treatments, including 25% benzyl benzoate emulsion, 0.5% malathion cream, 1% gamma benzene hexachloride (lindane) lotion, and 1% permethrin. In children benzyl benzoate should be diluted to 10% and used with care as toxicity results from absorption. In infants over 2 months old permethrin or 2.5% sulphur ointment can be used. Gamma benzene hexachloride should not be given to children under 10 or pregnant women in the first trimester. Important points are:

(1) The patient should wash well: a hot bath was formerly advocated but it is now known that this may increase absorption through the skin.

(2) The lotion should be applied from the neck down, concentrating on affected areas and making sure that the axillae, wrists, ankles, and pubic areas are included. If there is any doubt about the thoroughness of application the process should be repeated in a few days.

(3) All contacts and members of the patient's household should be treated at the same time.

(4) Residual papules may persist for many weeks. Topical steroids can be used to relieve the itching.

(5) Secondary infection as a result of scratching may need to be treated.

Demodex

Demodex folliculorum is a small mite that inhabits the human hair follicle, the eggs being deposited in the sebaceous gland. It is found on the central area of the face, chest, and neck of adults. It may have a role in the pathogenesis of rosacea, in which it may be found in large numbers. It may be associated with a pustular eruption round the mouth and blepharitis.

Larva migrans

The boy in the illustration had been on holiday at a coastal town in Kenya and regularly played on a beach frequented by dogs. Two weeks after returning to Britain he started itching on the buttocks and subsequently his parents noticed a linear, raised area that progressed to form a semicircle—a condition known as larva migrans, due to the larvae of the hookworm of dogs and cats, *Ancyclostoma caninum*. The ova are shed in the faeces and in a warm moist environment hatch into larvae that invade "dead end" hosts. They do not develop any further, so systemic disease does not occur.

Treatment—is either by freezing the advancing end of the lesion with liquid nitrogen or by applying thiabendazole (10%) suspension. Similar lesions in patients returning from tropical countries raises the possibility of larva migrans from strongyloides infestation, myiasis from the larvae of flies, or gnathostomiasis.

Visceral larva migrans caused by *Toxocara canis* and *Ascaris lumbricoides* may produce a transient rash.

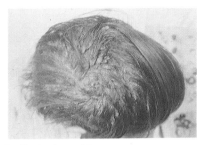

Pediculosis capitis.

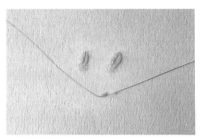

Head lice and nits.

Pediculosis (lice)

Infestation with lice became less common in the postwar years, but the incidence has recently increased.

There are three areas of the body usually affected by two species of wingless insects—*Pediculus humanus*, infecting the head and body, and *Phthirus pubis*, the pubic louse. The wingless insects feed on blood aspirated at the site of the bite, and each female lays 60–80 encapsulated eggs attached to hairs—"nits" in common parlance.

Head lice are transmitted via combs, brushes, and hats, being more common in girls than boys. The infestation is heaviest behind the ears and over the occiput. If the eyelashes of children are affected this is with "crab lice" (*Phthirus pubis*); it is not pediculosis.

Body lice are less common in western Europe. Transmission is by clothing and bedding, on which both lice and their eggs may be found in the seams. Poor hygiene favours infestation.

Pubic lice infestation occurs world wide and is generally transmitted by sexual contact. Infestation of eyelashes may occur with poor hygiene.

As a result of scratching there may be marked secondary infection that obscures the underlying infestation.

Treatment—Gamma benzene hexachloride 1% is usually effective as a single application. Permethrin can also be used.

Further reading

Alexander JO. *Arthropods and human skin.* Berlin: Springer-Verlag, 1984.
Busvine JR. *Insects and hygiene.* 3rd ed. London: Chapman and Hall, 1980.
Marshall AG. *The ecology of ectoparasitic insects.* New York: Academic Press, 1981.
Parish CL, Nutting WB, Schwartzman RM. *Cutaneus infestation of man and animal.* New York: Greenwood, 1983.

16. THE HAIR AND SCALP

Introduction

Hair, which has an essential physiological role in animals, is mainly of psychological significance in man. A good head of hair provides some degree of warmth for the human head and also protection from ultraviolet radiation, but its significance is otherwise in the eye of the beholder. In the form of wool, hair is of economic importance and considerable research has been carried out into the cycles of growth and the structure of wool keratin in sheep.

Too much hair, particularly on the face of women, is an embarassment and cosmetic problem and loss of hair from the scalp is equally troublesome. Changes in hair growth are not only of cosmetic significance but can also be associated with underlying diseases. Diseases occurring in the skin of the scalp can damage hair follicles leading to loss of hair.

This chapter covers:
(1) The normal pattern of hair growth.
(2) Causes of hair loss.
(3) Skin diseases involving the scalp.
(4) Causes of excess hair growth.
(5) Abnormalities of the hair itself.
(6) Treatment.

The normal pattern of hair growth

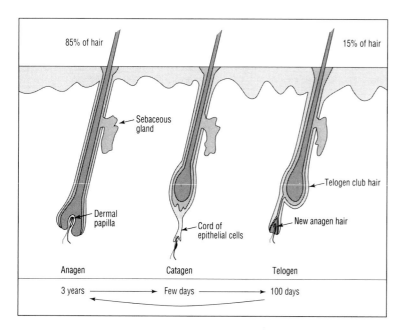

Unlike other epidermal structures which grow continuously, hair has a cyclical pattern of growth. The growing phase or *anagen* lasts an average of 1000 days on the scalp followed by an involutional phase known as *catagen* which is quite short, lasting only a few days. The hair then enters a resting phase, *telogen*, lasting about 100 days. In man, hair growth is normally asynchronous, with each individual hair following its own cycle independently of the others. The basal layer of the hair bulb from which the hair itself is produced is known as the matrix and contains melanocytes from which melanin pigment is incorporated into the hair. The type of melanin determines the colour and in grey or white hair, pigment production is reduced or absent.

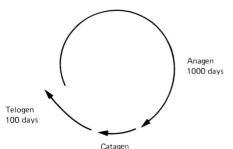

The body surface with the exception of the palms, soles, the lips, and the genitalia, is covered with fine vellus hairs that do not have a medulla and are not pigmented. These hairs develop into longer coarse, medullated, terminal hair on the scalp and eyebrows. At puberty a similar change occurs in the pubic area and the axillae, also on the face and trunk, in the male. These changes are androgen dependent, even in females, but testicular androgen is required to produce beard growth and balding in men.

Racial characteristics and the genetic make-up of the individual determine the type and colour of the hair. Straight black oriental hair is clearly different from the nordic blonde type.

Hair loss

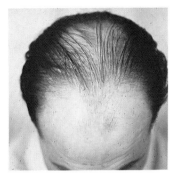

Male pattern baldness.

This is known as alopecia, derived from the Latin *Alopex*, a fox, presumably because of the bald patches of mange seen in wild foxes.

Adult male pattern alopecia is so common as to be considered normal. Circulating levels of testosterone are not raised in bald men but there is evidence that availability of the hormone to the hair follicle is increased. In postmenopausal women there may be widespread thinning of the hair but loss of hair at the temples often occurs to some degree at an earlier age.

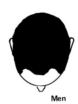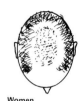

Men   Women

Alopecia may be *diffuse* or *localised*. If it is simply due to a physiological derangement of hair growth, the follicles remain intact, whereas inflammation may lead to scarring and loss of the hair follicles. Hence, hair loss can be classified into:

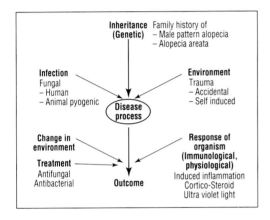

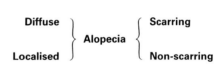

Diffuse hair loss

Causes of diffuse non-scarring alopecia

- Androgenetic alopecia
    - —male pattern
    - —female pattern
- Endocrine—thyroid disease (hypothyroidism and hyperthyroidism)
    - —hypopituitarism
    - —diabetes mellitus
- Stress —postpartum } telogen
    - —postoperative } effluvium
    - —postfebrile
- Drugs —cytotoxics
    - —anticoagulants } anagen
    - —antithyroid agents } effluvium
    - —cyclosporin
- Erythrodermic skin disease
    - —psoriasis
    - —eczema
    - —inflammatory
- Deficiency states
    - —protein malnutrition
    - —iron deficiency

An interuption of the normal hair cycle leads to generalised hair loss. This may be due to changes in circulating hormones, drugs, inflammatory skin disease, and "stress" of various types.

Telogen effluvium occurs if all the hairs enter into the resting phase together, most commonly after childbirth or severe illness. Two or three months later the new anagen hair displaces the resting telogen hair, resulting in a disconcerting, but temporary, hair loss from the scalp. Stress of any type, such as an acute illness or an operation, causes a similar type of hair loss.

Postfebrile alopecia occurs when a fever exceeds 39°C, particularly with recurrent episodes. It has been reported in a wide range of infectious diseases, including glandular fever, influenza, malaria, and brucellosis. It also occurs in fever associated with inflammatory bowel disease.

Dietary factors such as iron deficiency and hypoproteinaemia may play a role, but are rarely the sole cause of diffuse alopecia.

Severe malnutrition with a protein deficiency results in dystrophic changes with a reduction in the rate of hair growth.

Congenital alopecia—may occur in some hereditary syndromes.

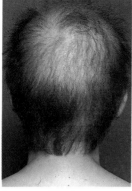

Anagen effluvium.

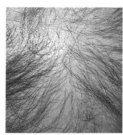

Diffuse alopecia caused by cyclosporin.

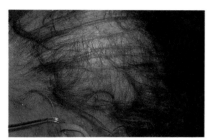

Diffuse alopecia caused by erythrodermic psoriasis.

Anagen effluvium occurs when the normal development of hair and follicle is interfered with, resulting in inadequate growth. As a result, hairs are shed earlier than usual, while still in the anagen phase.

Endocrine causes of diffuse alopecia include both hypo- and hyperthyroidism, hypopituitarism, and diabetes mellitus. In hypothyroidism the hair is thinned and brittle, whereas in hypopituitarism the hair is finer and soft but does not grow adequately.

Systemic drugs—Cytotoxic agents, anticoagulants, immunosuppressants, and some antithyroid drugs may cause diffuse hair—loss usually an "anagen effluvium" as mentioned above.

Inflammatory skin disease, when widespread, can be associated with hair loss, e.g. in erythroderma due to psoriasis or severe eczema.

Deficiency states are a rare cause of alopecia. Patients who suffer from hair loss are often convinced that there is some deviciency in the diet and may sometimes produce the results of an "analysis" of their hairs which show deficiencies in specific trace elements. In fact it is very difficult to cause actual hair loss even in gross malnutrition. Even in those dying from starvation in refugee camps, the hair growth in the scalp is usually present. In chronic malnutrition or kwashiorkor, the hair assumes a curious red/brown colour which may be due to iron deficiency.

Treatment

Wherever possible, the cause should be treated. This may be a matter of replacement therapy in hormonal deficiency. In alopecia due to stress once this cause is removed, hair growth may revert to normal. Treatment of inflammatory skin disease will result in some improvement of the hair loss.

Androgenic alopecia is best accepted, with assurance that it indicates normal virility.

Minoxidil lotion causes hair growth and is commercially available as a lotion. This has to be applied continuously every day as the scalp reverts to a level of loss which would have occurred without treatment as soon as it is stopped. It is effective in about half the patients with male pattern alopecia.

Localised alopecia

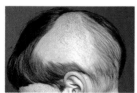

Alopecia areata.

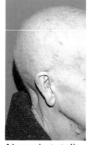

Alopecia areata, showing exclamation mark hairs.

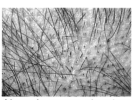

Alopecia totalis.

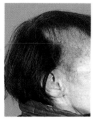

Trichotillomania.

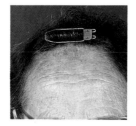

Traction alopecia.

Alopecia areata—This is a common form of hair loss. It is seen in 2% of patients attending the average dermatology clinic in the UK. There may be small patches of hair loss or the whole scalp may be affected. Resolution occurs in a few months or the condition may persist for years. There may be slight inflammation of the skin in the affected areas—in keeping with the possibility of an underlying immune reaction against the hair follicles. There is also an association with autoimmune disease and atopy.

In the affected areas the follicles are visible and empty. The hairs about to be lost have an "exclamation mark" appearance and in some areas that are resolving, fine vellus hairs are seen. Patches commonly occur on the scalp, face, or eyebrows. In *alopecia totalis*, the whole head is involved and in *alopecia universalis*, hair is lost from the whole of the body.

In many patients, particularly if it is a first episode, regrowth occurs within a few months with fine pale hairs appearing first, being replaced by normal adult hair. In older patients, non-pigmented hair may persist in previous patches of alopecia. Factors associated with a poor prognosis are:

(1) Repeated episodes of alopecia.
(2) Very extensive or complete hair loss (alopecia totalis).
(3) Early onset before puberty.
(4) In association with atopy.

Differential diagnosis includes trauma from the habit of plucking hair (trichotillomania) in mentally disturbed patients and traction alopecia from tight hair rollers or hair styles that involve tension on the hair. In fungal infections (tinea capitis) there is scaling and broken hairs. Fungal spores or hyphae are visible in hair specimens on microscopy.

Inflammation is present with loss of hair follicles in lupus erythematosis and lichen planus.

Treatment

An initial limited area of alopecia areata in adult life can be expected to regrow and treatment is generally not needed. Treatments that are carried out include:

(1) Injection of triamcinolone diluted with local anaesthetic which usually stimulates localised regrowth of hair. Unfortunately it often falls out again and there is a risk of causing atrophy. Topical steroid lotion can be used but results are variable.

(2) Ultraviolet light or PUVA can give good, if transient, results in a few patients but it has little effect in the majority. It may act by suppressing an immune reaction around the hair root.

(3) Induced contact dermatitis and irritants are occasionally effective. Cantharadin and dithranol have been used for many years as irritants. Primula leaves or chemicals (e.g. diphencyprone) can be applied to produce an acute contact dermatitis. The mechanism by which acute inflammation stimulates hair growth is not understood.

Aetiological factors in alopecia areata

- Genital — familial in about 20% of cases
  — associated with Down's syndrome
- Immunological — T lymphocytic infiltrate around hair follicles
  — associated with autoimmune disease
- Stress — may be associated in individual patients

Scarring alopecia

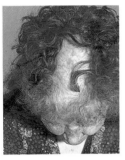

Systemic lupus erythematosus.

Causes of scarring alopecia

- Trauma — e.g. burns
- Inflammation
  - Acute — bacterial (pyogenic infection, syphilis)
    — viral (herpes simplex, herpes zoster, varicella)
    — fungal (kerion caused by animal ringworm)
  - Chronic — lupus erythematosus,
    — lichen planus
    — folliculitis decalvans
    — morphoea
  - Rare — pyoderma gangrenosum
    — necrobiosis lipoidica
    — sarcoidosis

En coup de sabre.

The absence of hair follicles is an important physical sign as it indicates:

(1) The presence of an inflammatory process that requires further investigation.

(2) That there is unlikely to be any significant recovery of hair growth.

The presence of inflammation does not necessarily produce marked erythema—in lichen planus and lupus erythematosus, the inflammatory changes are often chronic. Systemic lupus erythematosus produces areas of inflammation that extend, leaving residual scarring. In discoid lupus erythematosus there is more scaling with keratotic plugs in the follicle. Localised scleroderma (morphoea) also causes alopecia, often with a linear atrophic lesion—the *en coup de sabre* pattern.

More acute inflammatory changes are seen as a result of pyogenic infection or *kerion* in which there is a marked inflammatory reaction to fungal infection from cattle. In "folliculitis decalvans" there is florid folliculitis with deep-seated pustules and scarring. Treatment is with prolonged antibiotics.

Trauma can also cause scarring with alopecia.

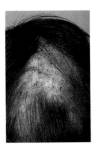

Folliculitis decalvans.

Skin disease involving the scalp

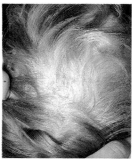

Tinea capitis.

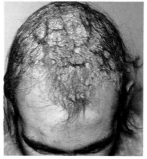

Pityriasis amiantacea.

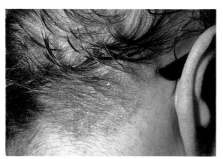

Contact eczema, hair dye.

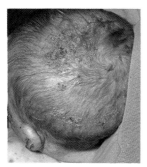

Atopic eczema.

Cutaneous diseases of the scalp

COMMON

- *Inflammatory*
  Psoriasis
  Seborrhoeic eczema
  Contact dermatitis

- *Infection*
  Folliculitis—staphylococcal or
  streptococcal
  Fungal infection
    microsporum, with hair loss
    trichophyton, with scaling and
      inflammation
  Herpes—zoster and simplex

- *Infestation*
  Pediculosis

LESS COMMON
  Lupus erythematosus
  Lichen planus
  Pemphigoid and pemphigus

The scalp can be involved in any skin disease, but most commonly in psoriasis and seborrhoeic eczema. A mild degree of scaling from accumulation in skin scales is so common as to be normal (dandruff). Increased accumulation of scales is seen in seborrhoeic dermatitis in which pityrosporum organisms may play a part. Sometimes masses of thick adherent scales develop, in *pityriasis amiantacea*, usually due to psoriasis. Eczema and contact dermatitis can also involve the scalp.

Treatment

Scaling and inflammatory changes can be improved with the use of sulphur and salicylic ointment. It is effective but messy and best applied at night. Tar preparations, oil of cade, and coconut oil in various formulations are all effective. Topical steroids can also be used to suppress inflammation.

Hair shaft abnormalities

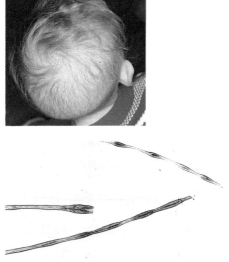

Monilethrix.

Congenital abnormalities of the hair shaft itself lead to weak, thin and broken hairs. In some cases there is a characteristic appearance, e.g. "spun glass" appearance of *pili torti* with a twisted hair. In *monilethrix* there are regular nodes in the hair shaft.

There are other abnormalities of the hair shaft which are not associated with increased fragility, such as the Willi hair syndrome, progressive kinking of the hair and uncombable hair in which the hair grows in disorderly profusion, completely resistant to combing and brushing. In *pili annulati* there may be a spangled appearance due to bright bands in the hair shaft.

Excessive hair

<table>
<tr><td>

Causes of hypertrichosis

- Congenital (rare)
- Acquired—porphyria
  hyperthyroidism
  anorexia nervosa
  some developmental defects,
     e.g. Hurler's syndrome
  tumours (hypertrichosis
     lanuginosa)
  drugs (diazoxide, minoxidil,
     cyclosporin)

</td></tr>
</table>

Causes of hirsutism	
• Hereditary, racial	
• Endocrine	
Adrenal	—virilising tumours Cushing's syndrome adrenal hyperplasia
Ovarian	—virilising tumours polycystic ovary syndrome
Pituitary	—acromegaly hyperprolactinaemia
• Iatrogenic	—anabolic steroids, androgens, corticosteroids, danazol, phenytoin, psoralens (in PUVA)

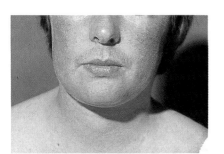

Hirsuties due to virilising tumour.

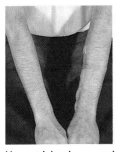

Hypertrichosis caused by minoxidil.

There are two types of overgrowth of hair:

(1) *Hirsuties* is the growth of coarse terminal hair in a male distribution occurring in a woman.

(2) *Hypertrichosis* is a generalised excessive growth of hair.

Hirsuties most commonly occurs after the menopause and may be present to some degree in normal women as a result of familial or racial traits. It may arise without any underlying hormonal disorder or as a result of virilising hormones. These causes are listed in the box on the left. In addition to androgens, a number of drugs can cause hirsuties. It is important to remember that hirsuties may be part of a virilising syndrome or polycystic ovaries. It is useful to measure the serum testosterone and oestrogen level, as well as urinary 17 oxosteroid concentrations.

Treatment

For idiopathic hirsuitism, treatment includes:

(*a*) Removal of hair by shaving or hair removing creams.

(*b*) Electrolysis and diathermy give permanent destruction of the hair follicle.

(*c*) Anti-androgen drugs such as cyproterone can be used under specialist supervision.

Further reading

Orfanos CE, Happle R. *Hair and hair disease.* Berlin: Springer-Verlag, 1990.
Rook A, Dawber R. *Diseases of the hair and scalp.* 3rd ed. Oxford: Blackwell Scientific, 1997.

17. DISEASES OF THE NAILS

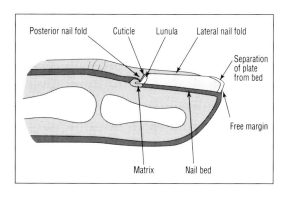

Posterior nail fold — Cuticle — Lunula — Lateral nail fold — Separation of plate from bed — Free margin — Matrix — Nail bed

In animals and birds claws are used for digging and grasping as well as for fighting. The human nail may be used as a weapon but its main function is to protect the distal soft tissues of the fingers and toes.

As an ectodermal derivative composed of keratin, the nail plate grows forward from a fold of epidermis over the nail bed which is continuous with the matrix proximally. The keratin composing the nail is derived mainly from the matrix with contributions from the dorsal surface of the nail fold and the nail bed also adds keratin to the deep surface.

The nail grows slowly for the first day after birth then more rapidly until it slows in old age. The rate of nail growth is greater in the fingers than the toes, particuly on the dominant hand. It is slower in women but increases during pregnancy. Finger nails grow at approximately 0·8 mm per week and toe nails 0·25 mm per week.

Physical signs in the nails

The changes in the nail may be due to a local disease process, a manifestation of a skin disease, or due to a systemic disorder. Hereditary disorders may also affect the nails. It is therefore important to take both a general history and specifically enquire about skin diseases. It sometimes happens that the nail changes are the only sign of a dermatological disease, although the patient may have a previous history of lichen planus or psoriasis, for example.

Localised infection or trauma will affect one or two nails. *Skin disease*, such as psoriasis, affects many or all nails, usually symmetrically, whereas *systemic illness* or drugs will affect all the nails.

Local nail changes

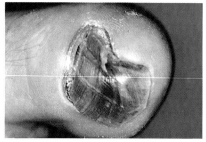

Trauma.

Trauma
- Acute trauma which may remove the whole nail.
- Chronic trauma as a result of badly fitting footwear which may cause thickening of the nail with deformed growth, *onychogryphosis*. Chronic trauma due to overenthusiastic manicuring or habitual picking at finger nails can result in deformity and impaired growth.
- Repeated trauma in occupations that involve repetitive action, such as assembling cardboard boxes. This may cause detachment of the nail (*onycholysis*) or splitting of the nails.

Infection
- Infection of the tissues around the nail (*paronychia*) is often mixed with pyogenic organisms, including *Pseudomonas*, as well as yeasts such as candida. This condition occurs most frequently in those employed in the food industry and occupations where there is repeated exposure to a moist environment and minor trauma. The index and middle fingers are most frequently involved.

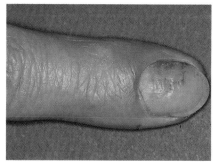

Paronychia.

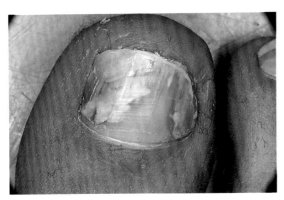

Fungal infection.

- Infection of the nail plate itself occurs in fungal infections which are comonly due to *Trichophyton* or *Epidermophyton* species.
- Those living in the tropics may acquire infection with *Scopulariopsis brevicaulis* which produces a black discoloration of the nail.

Skin diseases affecting the nails

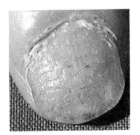

Pitting of nail.

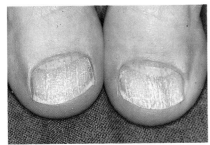

Lichen planus.

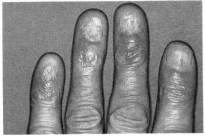

Dystrophy due to lichen planus.

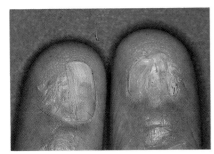

Pterygium formation.

Since the nail plate consists of specialised keratin produced by basal cells, it is not surprising that it is affected by skin diseases. Some conditions, such as psoriasis, may produce characteristic changes whereas in other conditions, such as eczema, the changes are much less specific.

Psoriasis causes an accumulation of keratin, as in lesions of the skin. This may result in the nail being both thickened and raised from the nail bed (*onycholysis*). There may be the changes of pustular psoriasis in the surrounding tissues, indistinguishable from acrodermatitis pustulosa. Loss of minute plugs of abnormal keratin results in "pitting".

Lichen planus produces atrophy of the nail plate which may completely disappear. The cuticle may be thickened and grow over the nail plate, known as *pterygium formation*.

Eczema may be associated with brittle nails that tend to split. Thickening and deformity of the nail occurs in eczema or contact dermatitis, sometimes with horizontal ridging.

Darrier's disease results in dystrophy of the nail and longitudinal streaks which end in triangular-shaped nicks at the free edge. On the skin there may be the characteristic brownish scaling papules on the central part of the back, chest, and neck. These are made worse by sun exposure.

Alopecia areata is quite often associated with changes in the nails including ridges, leuconychia and friable nails. It may be associated with '20 nail dystrophy'.

Auto-immune conditions such as pemphigus and pemphigoid may be associated with a variety of changes including ridging, splitting of the nail plate and atrophy in some or all of the nails.

Discoloration of the nail and friability are associated with *lupus erythematosus*.

Diseases of the nails

General diseases affecting the nails

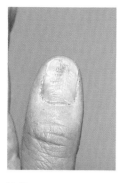

Nail dystrophy.

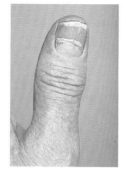

Beau's lines.

Nail changes in systemic illness—Acute illness results in a transverse line of atrophy known as a Beau's line. Shedding of the nail, *onychomedesis*, may occur in severe illness.

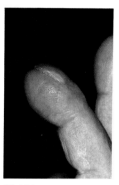

Clubbing.

Chronic diseases—Clubbing affects the soft tissues of the terminal phalanx with swelling and an increase in the angle between the nail plate and the nail fold. It is associated with chronic repiratory disease, cyanotic heart disease, and occasionally in chronic gastrointestinal conditions. It is occasionally hereditary and may be unilateral in association with vascular abnormalities.

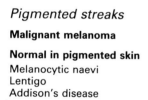

Pigmented streaks
Malignant melanoma
Normal in pigmented skin Melanocytic naevi Lentigo Addison's disease

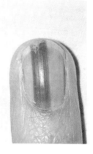

Colour changes—All the nails may be *white* due to hypoalbuminaemia in conditions such as cirrhosis of the liver. *Brown* discoloration is seen in renal failure and the "*yellow nail syndrome*" may be associated with abnormalities of the lymphatic drainage. The nail may have a *yellow* colour in jaundice. *Drugs* may cause changes in colour, e.g. tetracycline may produce *yellow* nails, antimalarials a blue discolouration, and chlorpromazine a *brown* colour. Leukonychia or whiteness of the nails occurs in fungal infections. Small white spots on the nail are quite commonly seen and are thought to be due to trauma of the nail plate.

Longitudinal pigmented streaks result from increased melanin deposition in the nail plate.

Longitudinal brown streaks are frequently seen in individuals with racially pigmented skin, particularly after trauma. This is rare in caucasians but occurs as a result of a benign pigmented naevus at the base of the nail and in associated lentigo. The most important cause to remember is *subungual melanoma* which may present with a longitudinal deep brown or black streak. Hutchinson's sign with pigmentation extends into the surrounding tissues, particularly the cuticle. Adrenal disease may rarely be associated with longitudinal streaks.

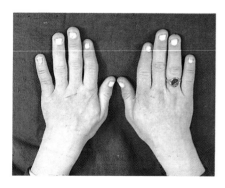

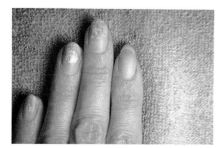

Leukonychia.

Specific changes in the nail plate

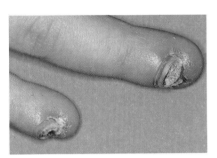

Psoriasis.

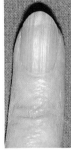

Psoriasis.

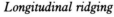

Onycholysis.

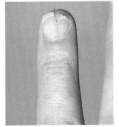

Darrier's disease.

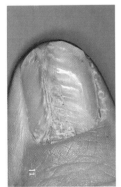

Longitudinal ridge.

Thickening

This may be due to:

- Hyperkeratosis
    psoriasis
    fungal infection
- Hypertrophy
    chronic trauma (onychogryphosis)
    pachyonychia congenita
- Atrophy
    lupus erythematosus
    lichen planus
    congenital dystrophy.

Thickening of the nail plate may be due to hyperkeratosis in psoriasis, in which case the changes will be symmetrical and there may well also be pitting of the nail and onycholysis. Similar changes are seen in fungal infection of the nail, which may be symmetrical on the toes. Nail clippings should be sent for microscopy and mycological culture.

Hypertrophy of the nail plate occurs as a result of chronic trauma, with only a few nails affected, and is usually seen in the feet. *Pachyonychia congenita* is a rare congenital disorder characterised by hypertrophic nails.

Hyperkeratosis, due to the accumulation of keratin under the nail plate, is also seen in psoriasis. It occurs occasionally in association with chronic dermatitis.

Detachment of the nail plate (onycholysis)

- Psoriasis
- Fungal infection
- Trauma
- Thyrotoxicosis.

Onycholysis is due to a detachment of the nail from the nail bed. If it is extensive, there may be complete loss of the nail plate. It is most commonly seen in psoriasis and occasionally in fungal infections of the nail. It may occur as a result of trauma or thyrotoxicosis.

Pitting of the surface of the nail plate

- Psoriasis
- Alopecia.

Pitting of the nail plate is due to punctate depressions on the surface of the nail plate. They are most often seen in psoriasis but may occur in alopecia areata.

Horizontal ridging

- Beau's lines following systemic illness and acute episodes of hand dermatitis.

Longitudinal ridging

- Single due to pressure from nail fold tumours
- Multiple due to lichen planus
- Alopecia areata
- Psoriasis
- Darrier's disease

Ridging represents a disturbance of nail growth. Inflammation as seen in acute paronychia or trauma can result in a single nail developing a horizontal ridge. Following an acute illness, there may be horizontal lines on all the nails.

A single longitudinal ridge can result from pressure due to benign or malignant tumours in the nail fold. A mucoid cyst can produce a longitudinal ridge. Multiple longitudinal lines are characteristic of lichen planus, psoriasis, alopecia areata, and Darrier's disease.

Koilonychia is a concave deformity of the nail plate, generally occurring in the finger nails. It may be idiopathic or occur as a result of iron deficiency anaemia.

Lesions adjacent to the nail

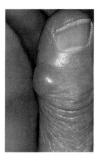

Mucoid cyst.

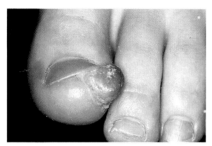

Big toe exostosis.

Mucoid cysts develop subcutaneously over the distal interphalangeal joint and may be adjacent to the nail, producing abnormalities of growth. These cysts develop as an extension of the synovial membrane and are linked to the joint by a fine tract. Very careful excision is required for a cure.

Naevi may occur adjacent to the nail and a benign melanocytic naevus can produce a pigmented streak. Subungual melanoma may produce considerable pigmentation of the nail and often causes pigmentation of the cuticle, so called Hutchinson's sign. Sometimes subungual melanoma is amelanotic so there is no pigmentary changes and any rapidly growing soft tumour should raise suspicions of this condition.

Subungual exostosis can cause a painful lesion under the nail. It is confirmed by X-ray films.

Glomus tumours arise as tender nodules.

Periungual fibrokeratomas also develop in patients with tuberous sclerosis.

Treatment of nail conditions

It is clearly not possible to treat congenital abnormalities of the nail, but avoiding exposure to trauma may help. Nail changes associated with dermatological conditions may improve as the skin elsewhere is treated. Systemic treatment of associated dermatoses will of course tend to improve the nail as well, e.g. methotrexate or retinoids for psoriasis.

Infective lesions respond to antifungal or antibiotic treatment. In chronic paronychia there is often a mixed infection and a systemic antibiotic combined with topical nystatin may be required. It is also important to keep the hands as dry as possible.

The imidazole antifungal drugs are fairly effective but are fungistatic. Terbinafine is fungicidal and a short course is as effective as prolonged treatment with the older drug griseofulvin.

Further reading
Baden HP. *Diseases of the hair and nails.* Chicago: Year Book Medical, 1986.
Baran R. *Nail disorders: common presenting signs, differential diagnosis and treatment.* Edinburgh: Churchill Livingstone, 1991.
De Berker DA, Baran R, Dawber RP. *Handbook of diseases of the nails and their management.* Oxford: Blackwell Scientific, 1995.

18. LUMPS AND BUMPS

The skin is a common site for neoplastic lesions, but most invade only locally and with treatment usually do not pose any threat to the life of the patient. The exception is malignant melanoma, which is dealt with in the next chapter. This is a rare tumour with a high mortality, and recent publicity campaigns have been aimed at preventing the tragedy of fatal metastases from a neglected melanoma.

As a result a large number of patients are being seen with pigmented skin lesions and nodules, only a very few of which are neoplastic. The question is how to distinguish the benign, the malignant, and the possibly malignant. The following guidelines may help in deciding whether the lesion can be safely left or should be treated.

A correlation of the clinical and pathological features is helpful in making a confident diagnosis of the more common tumours.

Seborrhoeic warts

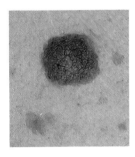 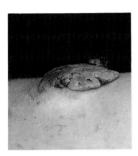

Seborrhoeic warts come in various shapes, sizes, and colours. When deeply pigmented, inflamed, or growing they may appear to have the features of a malignant lesion, but the following features are characteristic:
- Well defined edge.
- Warty, papillary surface—often with keratin plugs.
- Raised above surrounding skin to give a "stuck on" appearance.
Individual lesions vary considerably in size, but are usually 0·5–3 cm in diameter. Protuberant and pedunculated lesions occur. Solitary lesions are commonly seen on the face and neck but more numerous, large lesions tend to occur on the trunk. They become more common with increasing age.

Basal cell carcinoma

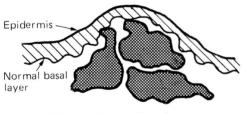

Epidermis

Normal basal layer

Nodular basal cell carcinoma

In contrast, the early basal cell carcinoma—or rodent ulcer—presents as a firm nodule, clearly growing within the skin and below it, rather than on the surface. The colour varies from that of normal skin to dark brown or black, but there is commonly a "pearly" translucent quality. As its name implies, the tumour is composed of masses of dividing basal cells that have lost the capacity to differentiate any further. As a result no epidermis is formed over the tumour and the surface breaks down to form an ulcer, the residual edges of the nodule forming the characteristic "rolled edge." Once the basal cells have invaded the deeper tissues the rolled edge disappears.

Ulcerated basal cell carcinoma

Ulcer with a rolled edge

Becomes

Clumps of neoplastic basal cells

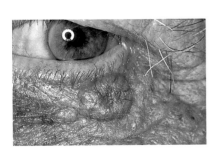 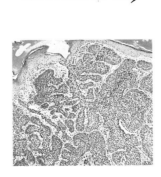 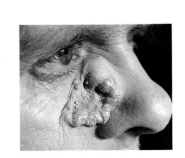

Lumps and bumps

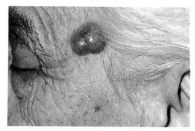

Cystic basal cell carcinoma.

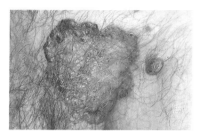

Superficial basal cell carcinoma.

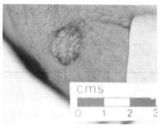

Pigmented basal cell carcinoma.

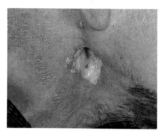

Neglected basal cell carcinoma (rodent ulcer).

Variants

Variants of the usual pattern can cause problems in diagnosis. *Cystic* basal cell carcinomas occur and those that show differentiation towards hair follicles or sweat glands may have a less typical appearance. *Pigmented* lesions can resemble melanoma. The *superficial spreading* type may be confused with a patch of eczema. This usually occurs on the trunk, does not itch, and shows a gradual but inexorable increase in size. A firm "whipcord" edge may be present.

Treatment

Various methods of destroying tumour tissue are used and the results are similar for radiotherapy and surgical excision:

(1) Ulcerated lesions may invade tissue planes, blood vessels, and nerves more extensively than is clinically apparent.

(2) Although modern techniques of radiotherapy result in minimal scarring and atrophy these may cause problems near the eye.

(3) Basal cell carcinomas in skin creases, such as the nasolabial fold, tend to ulcerate and are hard to excise adequately.

(4) Surgical excision has the advantage that should the lesion recur radiotherapy is available to treat it, whereas it is not desirable to treat recurrences after radiotherapy with further irradiation.

Squamous cell carcinoma

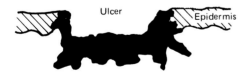

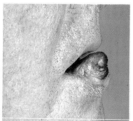

Squamous neoplastic cells

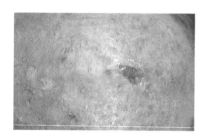

Squamous cell carcinoma represents proliferation of the epidermal keratinocytes in a deranged manner—with a visible degree of differentiation into epidermal cells that may show individual cell keratinisation and "pearls" of keratin. In other tumours bizarre cells with mitoses, cells with clear cytoplasm, or spindle cells may be seen.

This type of cancer often develops at a site of previous damage to the skin—for example, from sunlight or chemical damage. The first change clinically is a thickening of the skin with scaling or hyperkeratosis of the surfaces. The more differentiated tumours often have a warty, keratotic crust while others may be nodular. The edge is poorly defined. There may be associated dilated, telangiectatic blood vessels. The original hard, disc like lesion becomes nodular and ulcerates with strands of tumour cells invading the deeper tissue. The thick warty crust, often found elsewhere, may be absent from the lesions on the lip, buccal mucosa, and penis.

These histological changes complement the clinical appearance and are clearly different from those of basal cell carcinoma.

Treatment—Small lesions should be excised as a rule, making sure that the palpable edge of the tumour is included, with a 3–5 mm margin. Radiotherapy is effective but fragile scars may be a disadvantage on the hand. Cryotherapy or topical fluorouracil can be used for histologically confirmed, superficial lesions and also for solar keratoses.

Solar keratoses

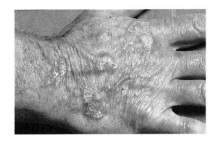

Squamous cell carcinoma may develop in solar keratoses, which show thickening of the epidermis and abnormal keratinocytes. They occur on sites exposed to the sun and are more common on those who have worked out of doors or sunbathed excessively. They can be regarded as squamous cell carcinomas grade 1/2 but do not necessarily progress to a dysplastic carcinoma. They also develop on the lips, particularly of pipe smokers.

The clinical appearance varies from a simple rough area of skin to a keratotic lesion with marked inflammation. The edge and surface are irregular.

Treatment with cryotherapy, using liquid nitrogen or carbon dioxide, repeated if necessary, is usually effective.

5-Fluorouracil cream is useful for larger or multiple lesions. It is applied twice daily for two weeks, which produces inflammation and necrosis. Simple dressings are applied for the next two weeks. This process can be repeated if necessary. As it is a cytotoxic drug it should be handled with care and applied sparingly with a cotton bud while wearing gloves.

Other conditions

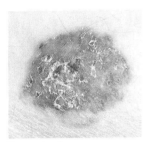

Bowen's disease.

Bowen's disease is characterised by a well defined, erythematous macule with little induration and slight crusting. It is a condition of the middle aged and elderly, occurring commonly on the trunk and limbs. It is an intraepidermal carcinoma, which has been reported to follow the ingestion of arsenic in "tonics" taken in years gone by or exposure to sheep dip, weedkiller, or industrial processes. After many years florid carcinoma may develop with invasion of deeper tissues. It may be confused with a patch of eczema or superficial basal cell carcinoma. Lesions on covered areas may be associated with underlying malignancy. Erythroplasia of Queyrat is a similar process occurring on the glans penis or prepuce.

Paget's disease of the nipple presents with unilateral non-specific erythematous changes on the aureola and nipple, spreading to the surrounding skin. The cause is an underlying adenocarcinoma of the ducts. It should be considered in any patient with eczematous changes of one breast that fail to respond to simple treatment. Extramammary lesions occur.

Keratoacanthoma is a rapidly growing fleshy nodule that develops a hard keratotic centre. Healing occurs with some scarring. Although benign, it may recur after being removed with curette and cautery, particularly from the face, and is best excised.

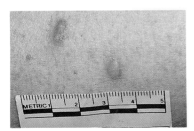

Paget's disease of the nipple.

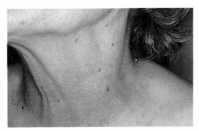

Keratoacanthoma.

Benign tumours

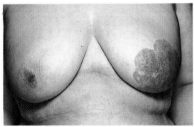

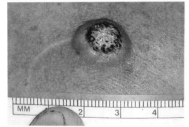

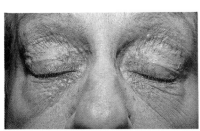

Dermatofibroma (top left), skin tags (above), and syringoma (left).

Dermatofibroma—This is a simple, discrete firm nodule, arising in the dermis at the site of an insect bite or other trivial injury. Often there is a brown or red vascular lesion initially which then becomes fibrotic—a sclerosing haemangioma. The histiocytoma is similar but composed of histiocytes.

Skin tags may be pigmented but rarely cause any diagnostic problems unless inflamed. Some are in fact pedunculated seborrhoeic warts and others simple papillomas (fibroepithelial polyps).

Other benign tumours

A wide variety of tumours may develop from the hair follicle and sebaceous, exocrine (sweat), and apocrine glands. The more common include *syringomas*—slowly growing, small, multiple nodules on the face of eccrine gland origin.

Lumps and bumps

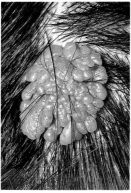

Naevus sebaceous.

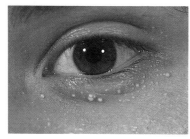

Verrucous epidermal naevus.

Naevus sebaceous is warty, well defined, varying in size from a small nodule to one several centimetres in diameter. Lesions occur in the scalp of children, may be present at birth, and gradually increase in size. They may proliferate or develop into a basal cell carcinoma in adult life and they are therefore best removed.

Verrucous epidermal naevi are probably a variant, found on the trunk and limbs.

Cysts

The familiar *epidermoid cyst*—also known as sebaceous cyst or wen—occurs as a soft, well defined, mobile swelling usually on the face, neck, shoulder, and chest. It is not derived from sebaceous glands but contains keratin produced by the lining wall.

Pilar cysts on the scalp are similar lesions derived from hair follicles.

Milia are small keratin cysts consisting of small white papules found on the cheek and eyelids.

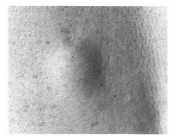

Epidermoid cyst.

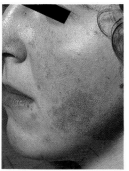

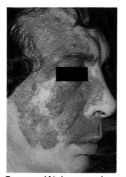

Milia.

Vascular lesions

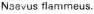

Naevus flammeus.

Sturge–Weber syndrome.

The more common vascular naevi are mentioned.

The port wine stain, or naevus flammeus, presents at birth as a flat red lesion, usually on the face, neck, or upper trunk. There is usually a sharp midline border on the more common unilateral lesions. In time the affected area becomes raised and thickened because of proliferation of vascular and connective tissue. If the area supplied by the ophthalmic or maxillary divisions of the trigeminal nerve is affected there may be associated angiomas of the underlying meninges with epilepsy—Sturge–Weber syndrome. Lesions of the limb may be associated with arteriovenous fistulae.

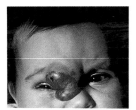

Cavernous angioma in a 5-month-old baby.

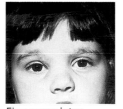

Five years later without treatment.

Cavernous angioma—strawberry naevi—appear in the first few weeks of life or at birth. A soft vascular swelling is found, most commonly on the head and neck. The lesions resolve spontaneously in time and do not require treatment.

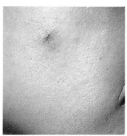

Spider naevi.

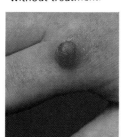

Pyogenic granuloma.

Spider naevus consist of a central vascular papule with fine lines radiating from it. They are more common in children and women. Large numbers in a man raise the possibility of liver disease.

Campbell de Morgan spots are discrete red papules 1–5 mm in diameter. They are more common on the trunk.

Pyogenic granuloma is a lesion that contains no pus but is in fact vascular and grows rapidly. It may arise at the site of trauma. Distinction from amelanotic melanoma is important.

Further reading

Enzinger F, Weiss S. *Soft tissue tumours.* 2nd ed. St Louis: Mosby, 1988.
Mackie RM. *Skin cancer: an illustrated guide to the etiology, clinical features, pathology and management of benign and malignant cutaneous tumours.* 2nd ed. London: Martin Dunitz, 1996.

19. BLACK SPOTS IN THE SKIN

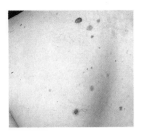
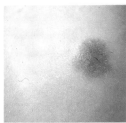

There has been a great increase in public awareness of melanoma and any dark lesions of the skin are sometimes regarded with the same dread as Long John Silver's "black spot" in *Treasure Island*—a sign of imminent demise. However, the vast majority of pigmented lesions are simply moles or harmless pigmented naevi. The most important thing is to know which moles can be safely ignored and which should be removed. Benign moles are described first, then malignant melanoma, followed by a discussion of the differences between these two.

Benign moles

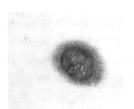

Benign pigmented naevi.

Benign moles are naevi with a proliferation of melanocytes and a variable number of dermal naevus cells. Most develop in early childhood and adolescence. The number of moles remains constant during adult life with a gradual decrease from the sixth decade onwards.

There is often an increase in both the number of moles and the degree of pigmentation during pregnancy.

Acquired melanocytic naevi

Acquired melanocytic naevi are the familiar moles and present in a number of different ways depending on the type of cells and the depth in the skin.

Junctional naevi are flat macules with melanocytes proliferating along the dermo-epidermal border.

Compound naevi have pigmented naevus cells at the dermo-epidermal border and in the dermis, producing a raised brown lesion. The dermal melanocytes may accumulate around the skin appendages and blood vessels and form a band of cells without melanin or more deeply penetrating strands of spindle cells. Proliferating naevus cells may throw the overlying epidermis into folds, giving a papillary appearance.

In a purely *intradermal naevus* the junctional element is lost, with the deeper cells showing characteristics of neural tissue. Other types of acquired pigmented naevi include:

Blue naevus—This is a collection of deeply pigmented melanocytes situated deep in the dermis, which accounts for the deep slate-blue colour.

Spitz naevus—This presents as a fleshy pink papule in children. It is composed of large spindle cells and epitheloid cells with occasional giant cells, arranged in "nests". It is benign and the old name of juvenile melanoma should be abandoned.

Halo naevus—This consists of a melanocytic naevus with a surrounding halo of depigmentation associated with the presence of antibodies against melanocytes in some cases. The whole naevus gradually fades in time.

Becker's naevus—This is an area of increased pigmentation, often associated with increased hair growth, which is usually seen on the upper trunk or shoulders. It is benign.

Freckles or ephelides—These are small pigmented macules, less than 0·5 cm in diameter, that occur in areas exposed to the sun in fair skinned people then fade during the winter months.

Dysplastic naevus syndrome—Multiple pigmented naevi occur, predominantly on the trunk, becoming numerous during adolescence. They vary in size—many being over 0·5 cm—and tend to develop malignant melanoma, particularly if there is a family history of this condition.

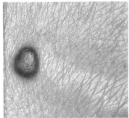

Blue naevus.

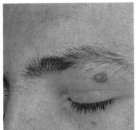

Spitz naevus.

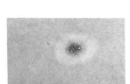

Halo naevus.

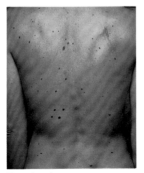

Dysplastic naevus syndrome.

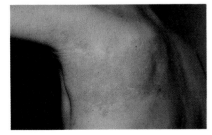

Becker's naevus.

Black spots in the skin

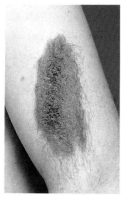

Congenital hairy naevus.

Congenital pigmented naevi

Congenital pigmented naevi are present at birth, generally over 1 cm in diameter, and vary from pale brown to black in colour. They often become hairy and more protuberant, possibly with an increased risk of malignant change. Larger lesions can cover a considerable area of the trunk and buttocks, such as the bathing trunk naevi, and their removal may present a considerable problem.

Melanoma

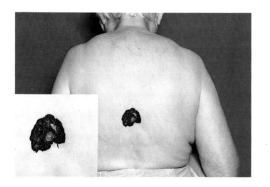

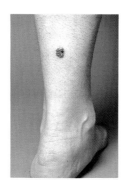

Melanoma is an invasive malignant tumour of melanocytes. Most cases occur in white adults over the age of 30, with a predominance in women.

Incidence—The incidence of melanoma has doubled over the past 10 years in Australia (currently 40/100 000 population) and shown a similar increase in other countries. In Europe twice as many women as men develop melanoma—about 12/100 000 women and 6/100 000 men.

Prognosis—The prognosis is related to the thickness of the lesion, measured histologically in millimetres from the granular layer to the deepest level of invasion. Lesions less than 0·76 mm thick have a 100% survival at five years, 0·76–1·5 mm thick an 80% survival at five years, and lesions over 3.5 mm less than 40% survival. These figures are based on patients in whom the original lesion had been completely excised. A recent study in Scotland has shown an overall five year survival of 71·6–77·6% for women and 58·7% for men.

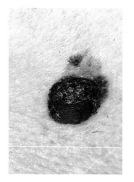

Nodular melanoma.

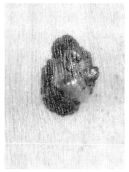

Superficial melanoma with nodules.

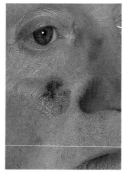

Lentigo maligna.

Sun exposure—The highest incidence of melanoma occurs in countries with the most sunshine throughout the year. However, skin type and the regularity of exposure to sun are also important. The incidence is much greater in fair skinned people from higher latitudes who have concentrated exposure to sun during holidays than those with darker complexions who have more regular exposure throughout the year. Severe sunburn may also predispose to melanoma.

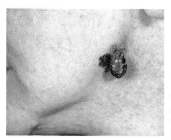

Nodule developing in superficial spreading melanoma.

Genetic factors—Since melanin protects the skin from ultraviolet light it is not surprising that melanoma occurs most commonly in fair skinned people who show little tanning on exposure to sun, particularly those of celtic origin. Members of families with the dysplastic naevus syndrome are more likely to develop melanoma in their moles. These patients have multiple naevi from a young age.

Pre-existing moles—It is rare for ordinary moles to become malignant but congenital naevi and multiple dysplastic naevi are more likely to develop into malignant melanoma.

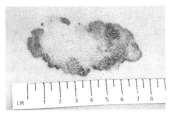

Superficial spreading
melanoma.

Types of melanoma

There are four main types of melanoma.

Superficial spreading melanoma is the more common variety. It is common on the back in men and on the legs in women. As the name implies the melanoma cells spread superficially in the epidermis, becoming invasive after months or years. The margin and the surface are irregular with pigmentation varying from brown to black. There may be surrounding inflammation and there is often clearing of the central portion. The invasive phase is associated with the appearance of nodules and increased pigmentation. The prognosis is correspondingly poor.

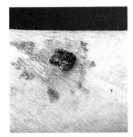

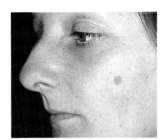

Nodular melanoma
in a lentigo.

Benign lentigo.

Lentigo maligna melanoma occurs characteristically in areas exposed to sun in elderly people. Initially there is a slowly growing, irregular pigmented macule that is present for many years before a melanoma develops.

Nodular melanoma presents as a dark nodule from the start without a preceding in situ epidermal phase. It is more common in men than women and is usually seen in people in their 50s and 60s. Because it is a vertical invasive growth phase from the beginning there is a poor prognosis.

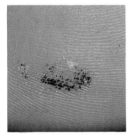

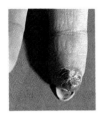

Acral melanoma.

Talon noir.

Acral melanoma occurs on the palm and soles and near or under the nails. Benign pigmented naevi may also occur in these sites and it is important to recognise early dysplastic change by using the criteria set out below. A very important indication that discoloration of the nail is due to melanoma is Hutchinson's sign—pigmentation of the nail fold adjacent to the nail. It is important to distinguish *talon noir*, in which a black area appears on the sole or heel. It is the result of trauma—for example, sustained while playing squash—causing haemorrhage into the dermal papillae. Paring the skin gently with a scalpel will reveal distinct blood filled papillae, to the relief of doctor and patient alike.

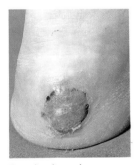

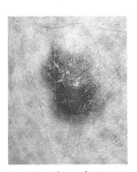

Dysplastic melanoma.

Amelanotic melanoma.

Other types of melanoma—As the melanoma cells become more dysplastic and less well differentiated they lose the capacity to produce melanin and form an *amelanonitic melanoma*. Such non-pigmented nodules may be regarded as harmless but are in fact extremely dangerous.

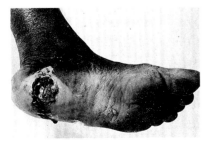

Malignant melanoma in a black person. Note the surrounding "halo".

How to tell the difference

Criteria for suspecting malignant changes in pigmented lesions

(1) *Growth*—Benign pigmented naevi continue to appear in adolescents and young adults. Any mole increasing in size in an adult over the age of 30 may be a melanoma

(2) *Shape*—Moles usually have a symmetrical, even outline, any indentations being quite regular; melanomas usually have an irregular edge with one part advancing more than the others

(3) *Colour*—Variation in colour of benign moles is even but a melanoma may be intensely black or show irregular coloration varying from white to slate blue, with all shades of black and brown. Inflammation may give a red colour as well. The amelanotic melanoma shows little or no pigmentation

(4) *Size*—Apart from congenital pigmentation naevi most benign moles are less than 1 cm in diameter. Any lesion growing to over 0·5 cm should be carefully checked

(6) *Itching*—Normally a mole does not itch but a melanoma may. Irritated seborrhoeic warts also itch

(7) *Bleeding* and crusting occur in an actively growing melanoma

If more than two of these features are present refer the patient for specialist opinion

A simple summary:

A—**A**symmetry of the lesion   B—Irregularity of the **B**order
C—Variations in **C**olour   D—**D**iameter larger than 0·5 cm

---

Benign moles show little change and remain static for years. Any change may indicate that a mole is in fact a melanoma or that a mole is becoming active. Size, shape, and colour are the most significant features and it is *change* in them that is most important. Patients with moles should have these changes explained to them, in particular that they indicate activity of the cells, not necessarily malignant change.

The sun and the skin

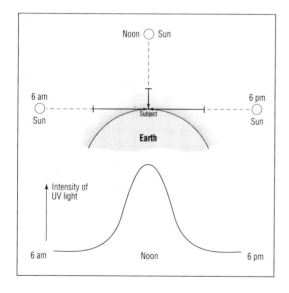

There is general awareness that the sun causes cancer in the skin with some people becoming obsessively fearful of any exposure to sun. A sensible approach with emphasis on reasonable precautions is called for. Useful points are:

- The non-melanotic, epidermal cancers—basal cell and squamous cell carcinomas—grow slowly and are not life threatening. Exposure to sun has usually occurred many years previously
- Most moles are entirely harmless
- Detecting the changes in moles or early melanoma, as outlined above, enables the diagnosis to be made at an early stage with a good chance of curative treatment
- Good sunscreen preparations should be used when outside in strong sunlight
- Reflected sun from the sea or beach can be nearly as damaging as direct sunlight
- Exposure to midday sun, particularly in tropical or subtropical latitudes, should be avoided. At this time the sunlight passes vertically through the atmosphere and there is less filtering of dangerous ultraviolet light.

Further reading

Ackerman AB. *Malignant melanoma and other melanocytic neoplasms.* Baltimore: Williams & Wilkins, 1984.
Roses DF. *Diagnosis and management of cutaneous malignant melanoma.* Philadelphia: Saunders, 1983.
Seigler HF. *Clinical management of melanoma.* The Hague: Nijhoff, 1982.

20. PRACTICAL PROCEDURES—HOW TO DO THEM AND WHERE TO USE THEM

Skin lesions are easily accessible for removal or biopsy and this needs to be appropriate to the site and type of lesion involved. It is important also to keep scarring to a minimum.

Destruction of skin lesions is carried out with:
Electrocautery
Cryotherapy
Laser treatment.

This is suitable for lesions where the diagnosis is certain, as no specimen is available for histology.

Removal of skin lesions results in a specimen for the pathologist to examine. The techniques used are:
Curettage and cautery
Surgical excision
Incisional biopsy which provides a specimen for histology to supplement the clinical diagnosis.

Cryotherapy

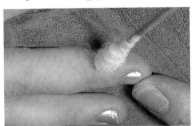

Applying the liquid nitrogen.

This involves the destruction of tissues by extreme cold. Current methods used are.

Carbon dioxide—Solid carbon dioxide (temperature $-79°C$) is produced by allowing rapid expansion of the compressed gas from a cylinder. This can be mixed with acetone to form a slush that can be applied with a cotton wool bud. A solid carbon dioxide stick, for direct application to lesions, is produced by an apparatus using "sparklet" bulbs.

The lesion must be frozen solid with a 1–2 mm margin of surrounding tissue. After thawing the freezing cycle should be repeated.

Liquid nitrogen ($-196°C$)—This can be simply applied using a cotton wool bud dipped in the vacuum flask of liquid nitrogen. Freezing takes a little longer than using spray apparatus. Various types of such apparatus are available with different sizes of nozzle. The larger ones are used for seborrheoic keratoses on the back, for example, and the smaller sizes for small lesions on the face. Freezing takes a few seconds and after thawing a further application can be made if necessary.

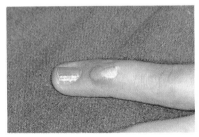

The frozen wart.

Ethyl chloride—This is sprayed directly on the skin, producing lowering of the temperature and temporary analgesia. It is not generally used for treatment.

Nitrous oxide—A cylinder of compressed gas is used to cool a probe to approximately $-80°C$. It is usually used for the treatment of warts and requires a 30-second freezing cycle.

Precautions

(1) Cryotherapy produces pain and inflammation. Blistering and sometimes haematoma can occur. This can be diminished by the application of a strong steroid cream immediately after freezing, but this should not be used for viral warts as it tends to encourage their proliferation.

(2) Damage to deeper structures is rare unless freezing of the deeper tissues is used; e.g. treating basal cell carcinoma.

(3) Accidental involvement of adjacent structures can occur particularly with the liquid nitrogen spray, so it is essential to screen them adequately. This applies particularly when carrying out freezing on the face, so avoid accidental spraying of the eye.

Skin lesions suitable for freezing

Viral warts—These may require several treatments at 2–3-week intervals.

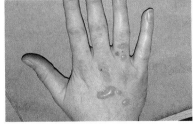

Subsequent slight blistering.

Practical procedures

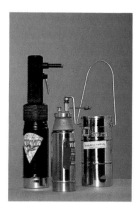
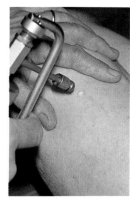

Practical points

(1) Be sure of the diagnosis before cryotherapy, taking a biopsy if necessary
(2) Explain to the patient that inflammation, blistering or haematoma formation may occur
(3) Use freezing with care on areas where the skin is thin, e.g.:
    (a) on the face and on children
    (b) on pigmented skin where postinflammatory hyperpigmentation can occur

Seborrhoeic keratoses—This responds well to cryotherapy, but as they are superficial lesions care must be taken to avoid excessive freezing with resultant scars.

Papillomata and skin tags—These can be easily and permanently treated by compression with artery forceps dipped in liquid nitrogen. Surprisingly, this is generally a painless procedure.

Dysplastic lesions—These lesions, which are potentially neoplastic or of low grade malignancy, can be effectively treated. This includes *solar keratoses*, if early and superficial, but follow-up is essential. The lesions can progress to squamous carcinoma and if not responding to cryotherapy should immediately be excised or removed with curettage and cautery for histological examination.

Bowen's disease—An intraepidermal carcinoma, if confirmed by incisional biopsy, can respond to repeated cryotherapy. Follow-up is essential.

Basal cell carcinoma—The superficial spreading type can be treated with liquid nitrogen but repeated and often prolonged freezing is required. Excision is often the preferred treatment. Nodular or invasive basal cell carcinomas can only be treated with deeper freezing with the use of a thermocouple probe to record the temperature at the base of the tumour to ensure complete destruction. This is not usually a routine procedure in general practice or outpatients.

Laser treatment

Laser—**L**ight **A**mplification by **S**timulated **E**mission of **R**adiation—produces high energy radiation. The first laser apparatus was developed from microwave technology in 1960 by the nobel prize winner T. H. Mamian. It was initially used as a destructive tool to ablate tumours but now different wavelengths can be directed at specific targets. Blood vessels, for example, take up the blue/green light of the argon laser and the red light of a ruby laser is well absorbed by the green dye of tattoos. Modern developments have resulted in laser equipment that produces minimal scarring and maximum specificity.

Although smaller portable units are available, laser treatment should still only be undertaken by those with appropriate training. The following are the skin lesions most commonly treated by laser.

Vascular lesions

Port wine stains—Argon and carbon dioxide lasers cause scarring, so yellow light omitting types such as Krypton, Flashlamp Powered Dye Laser (FPDL) or Copper Laser are used.

Telangiectasias—This is also treated with the FPDL, although this can cause transient purpura or copper laser.

Cavernous haemangioma—These can be treated by yellow dye laser followed by surgical excision.

Tattoos

Tattoos contain a variety of pigments so that more than one type of laser may be necessary for complete removal. The same pigment may vary in response in different patients. Superficial dark pigment usually responds to the Q switch ruby laser but deeper pigment may require the Nd:YAG laser or Alexandrite laser. Green pigment is usually removed with a Q switch ruby laser and red pigment with a green light laser such as the Q switch Nd:YAG. It is found that amateur tattoos are usually more easily removed than the professional type.

Pigmented lesions

Melanin absorbs light over a wide range of wavelengths, which can result in undesirable loss of skin colour following laser treatment. This can be put to good use in the treatment of benign lentigines and *café au lait* patches or deeply seated pigmented naevi. A wide range of laser types can be used, including Q switch ruby and Nd:YAG lasers. Congenital pigmented naevi should not be treated unless the biopsy has confirmed that they are benign.

Laser surgery

Lasers can be used as a cutting tool and recent studies have shown them to be a very effective means of producing incisions in the skin.

Electrocautery

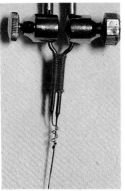
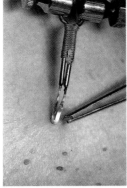

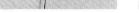

Pinpoint cautery attachment.

There are two forms of treatment:

(1) Heat from an electrically heated element, which is used for removal of skin tags and for treatment of the surface after curettage of warts, also seborrhoeic keratoses.

(2) High energy, low current "electrodesiccation" equipment which produces a high energy spark that can coagulate blood vessels or destroy some more papillomas. A fine needle point should be used for small telangiectatic naevi or milia. A larger needle is used for larger surfaces, e.g. after curettage.

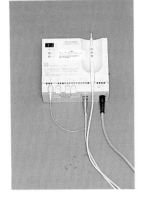
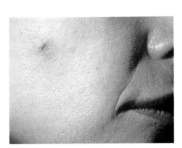

Blanch the lesion to identify feeding vessels. Then insert needle into feeding vessels in the cold state.

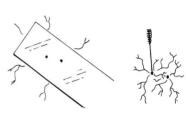

Curettage

This is a simple way of removing epidermal lesions. A curette has a metal spoon shaped end with a sharp cutting edge. There are a variety of shapes and sizes suitable for different lesions, from large seborrhoeic keratoses or papillomas to smaller ones for minute keratin cysts. A specimen is provided for histology but completeness of removal cannot be accurately assessed.

Local anaesthetic is used and, with the skin stretched, the curette is applied at the edge of the lesion which is then scooped off. It is advisable to work around the edges of larger or more firmly attached lesions. The dermis normally feels firm but when curetting off a keratotic

horn or solar keratoses, a soft consistency may indicate dysplastic change. The base can be lightly cauterised to control bleeding, sterilise the site, and prevent recurrence.

Small nodular basal cell carcinomas can be removed with curettage and cautery but the process should be repeated to remove as much abnormal tissue as possible and the scar should be inspected for possible recurrences after healing has occurred.

Various types of disposable curettes are available and are easy to use.

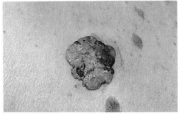
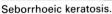

Seborrhoeic keratosis.

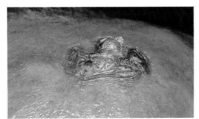

Actinic keratosis.

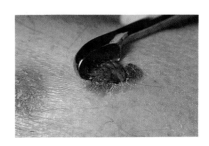

Lesions suitable for curetting

(1) Seborrhoeic keratoses
(2) Solitary viral warts
(3) Solar keratoses
(4) Cutaneous horns
(5) Small basal cell carcinomas

Curettage and cautery

(1) Use a sharp curette of appropriate size
(2) Very firm control of the curette prevents it from suddenly skidding onto normal skin
(3) Repeat curettage and cautery for neoplastic lesions such as basal cell carcinoma and solar keratoses

Incisional biopsy and punch biopsy

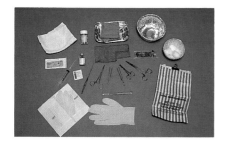

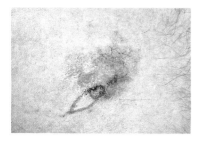

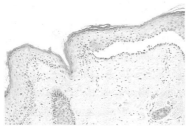

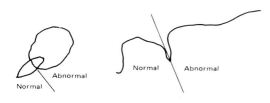

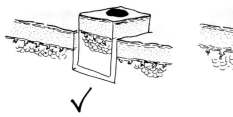

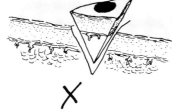

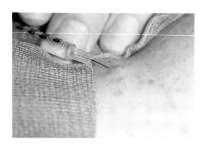

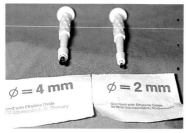

It is essential to have a working clinical diagnosis, but wherever there is doubt the pathologists can provide much more precise information regarding the nature and extent of the lesion. For example, a patch of Bowen's disease (intraepidermal carcinoma) may resemble sclerosing superficial basal cell carcinoma and a biopsy will usually distinguish them. Similarly, what appears to be a dysplastic pigmented naevus clinically may, on the one hand, prove to be benign or, on the other hand, turn out to be a malignant melanoma requiring wide excision.

Immunofluorescent staining of a blistering lesion differentiates dermatitis herpetiformis, which is treated with a gluten free diet, from pemphigoid, which requires corticosteroids and often immunosuppressant drugs.

Incisional biopsy—This is suitable for larger lesions and is taken across the margin of the lesion in the form of an elipse. It is essential to include deeper dermis, as the essential changes in, for example, granuloma or lymphoid infiltrate may not be near the surface. An adequate amount of normal tissue should be included, so this could be compared with the pathological area and this also means there is enough normal skin to suture the incision together.

Punch biopsy—The biopsy tool consists of a small cylinder with a cutting rim which is used to penetrate the epidermis by rotation between the operator's finger and thumb. There is minimal danger of damaging deeper structures as the elastic subcutaneous tissues merely rotate with the tool without being cut. The resulting plug of skin is lifted out with forceps and cut off as deeply as possible. The residual defect is treated with electrocautery.

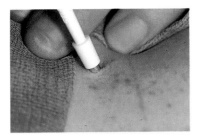
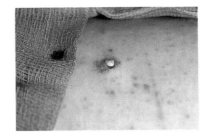
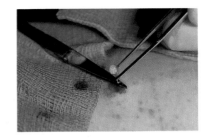

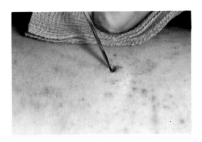
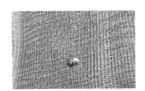

With the smaller sized punches the resulting defect can be treated with electrocautery or left to heal spontaneously. With a punch larger than 3 or 4 mm a single suture can be used. The main disadvantage of a punch biopsy is that it only provides a single small piece of tissue. It may not be representative or may miss an area of significant change. It tends to leave a more prominent scar than the incisional biopsy.

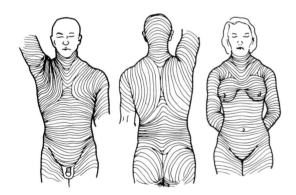

Excision of skin lesions is both curative and diagnostic. It may be the best way of making a diagnosis if there are multiple small papules or vesicles, one of which can be excised intact.

In the case of malignant lesions it is particularly important that the whole lesion is adequately excised.

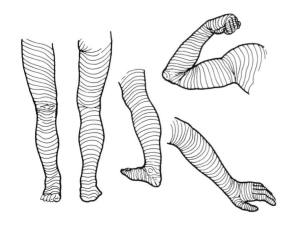
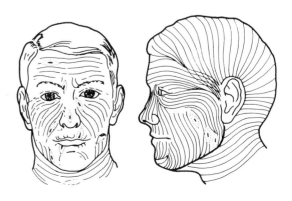

Practical procedures

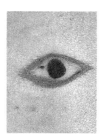

Clinical.

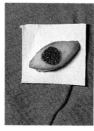

Surgical.

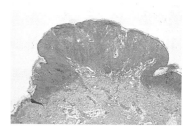

Histopathological.

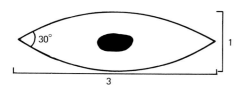

Surgical excision

(1) After initially inserting the needle, withdraw the plunger of the syringe to check the needle has not entered the blood vessels. Raising a small "bleb" of local anaesthetic ahead of the needle points helps to prevent this

(2) It is important to learn appropriate suturing techniques for different sites of the body and size of lesion

(3) Warn the patient that a scar will result and make sure that this is minimal and does not produce any deformity such as displacement of the eyelid.

(4) Always send an excised lesion for histology. A significant number of lesions diagnosed as being benign clinically excised outside dermatology units have been shown to be malignant. This would of course be missed if they had not been sent to a laboratory

Technique

The basic technique consists of making an eliptical incision with the length three times the width. This enables suturing without the formation of "dog ears" at the end. The long axis of the excision should follow the "wrinkle lines" of the skin, not the deeper lines of fascial attachment of Lange.

Lesions on the sternal area, upper chest and shoulders, where keloid scars often form, should only be excised when it is essential and may be best referred to a plastic surgeon.

Local anaesthetic is injected subcutaneously but close to the skin. The incision should be vertical rather than wedge shaped. Monofilament sutures cause less inflammation and trapping of serum than the braided variety, but are harder to tie.

Methods of suturing and the more specialised techniques of flaps and grafts are outside the scope of this book. Courses on minor surgery are generally available and there is no reason why any medical practitioner should not become fully competent in the handling of basic minor surgical techniques.

Further reading

Lawrence C. *Introduction to Dermatological Surgery.* Oxford: Blackwell Science, 1997.
Tromovitch TA, Stegman SJ, Glogau RG. *Flaps and grafts in dermatologic surgery.* Chicago: Year Book Medical, 1989.
Zachary CB. *Basic cutaneous surgery: a primer in technique.* New York: Churchill Livingstone, 1991.

21. IMMUNOLOGY AND THE SKIN

Types of allergic reaction

Type I - Immediate hypersensitivity

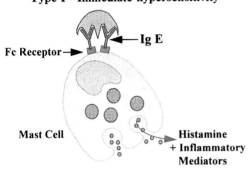

Fc Receptor →

Ig E

Mast Cell

Histamine
+ Inflammatory
Mediators

Type II - Cytotoxic

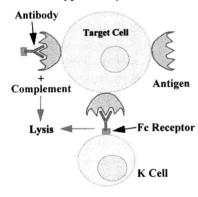

Antibody

Target Cell

+
Complement

Antigen

Lysis ←

Fc Receptor

K Cell

Type III - Circulating immune complexes

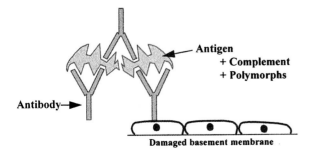

Antigen
+ Complement
+ Polymorphs

Antibody→

Damaged basement membrane

The skin has been described as the "immunological battleground of the body", so that reactions may occur in the skin rather than involving internal organs, e.g. an acute vasculitis occurring in the skin is unpleasant and requires treatment but the same reaction occurring in the kidneys can be life threatening. The immune response of the skin is used clinically in detecting the level of immunity to tuberculosis in the tuberculin skin test. It is also the means of immunisation where an injection of inactivated organisms induces an immune response but protects the entire body.

The different types of immune reaction are all manifested in the skin as part of a normal response to pathogens or as an allergic reaction. The difference is expressed by the word "allergy", first used by Von Pirquet in 1906, derived from the Greek ($\alpha\lambda o\zeta\ \varepsilon\nu\gamma o\nu$) meaning literally "other work". In other words it is a response that is appropriate for pathogenic organisms such as a tubercle bacillus but is misdirected against a harmless substance such as a rubber glove or the metal of a watch strap buckle.

There are three responses mediated by antibodies known as the *humoral* response and one by lymphocytes known as the *cell mediated* response.

(1) *Immediate hypersensitivity*—This type of reaction is caused by "reagin" antibodies, which are now known to consist mainly of IgE, that cause an acute anaphylactic reaction (without protection), which results in the release of histamine and vasoactive amines. Fortunately such reactions are rare but may occur in response to wasp stings and occasionally drug reactions. Severe reactions cause shock made worse by stress and exercise. A case was reported of a young woman who had a wasp sting when picnicking by a lake. She then plunged into the cold water, swimming vigorously, leading to a fatal anaphylactic reaction.

(2) *Cytotoxic reactions*—In this case cells become the target of attack by circulating antibodies with the involvement of complement. This may be caused by drugs or proteins attached to the cell surface that act as haptens so they become antigenic. They may also be destroyed by killer 'K' cells. A typical example is haemolytic anaemia.

(3) *Antigen–antibody complex reactions*—As a result of antibody production to antigens in the circulation, complexes form in the blood and these may be deposited in capillaries resulting in inflammatory changes. This involves the activation of complement and the release of mediators of inflammation producing vasodilatation and the accumulation of polymorphs.

Type IV - Delayed hypersensitivity

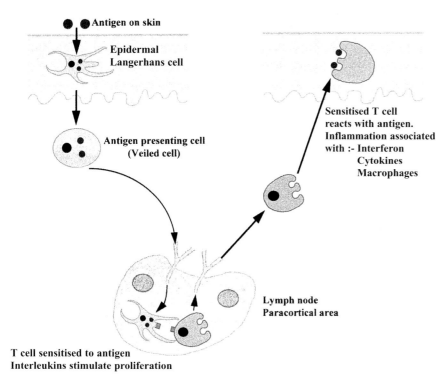

Antigen on skin

**Epidermal
Langerhans cell**

**Antigen presenting cell
(Veiled cell)**

**Sensitised T cell
reacts with antigen.
Inflammation associated
with :- Interferon
Cytokines
Macrophages**

**Lymph node
Paracortical area**

**T cell sensitised to antigen
Interleukins stimulate proliferation**

(4) *Delayed hypersensitivity*—This reaction results from lymphocytes known as T cells, because of their derivation from the thymus, which react with antigen in the skin. The reaction is initiated by antigen attached to Langerhan's cells in the epidermis being transported to the paracortical area of the regional lymph node with the production of lymphocytes sensitised specifically for that antigen. There is also the production of interleukin which has a feedback effect in stimulating the production of more sensitised lymphocytes. The reaction of the T lymphocytes in the epidermis results in the accumulation of macrophages and the release of inflammatory mediators.

Autoimmune disease and the skin

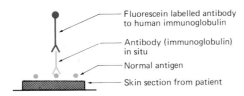

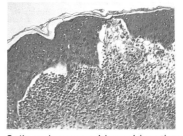

Split at dermatoepidermal junction.

There is always the risk that the well developed human immune system may react against the body's own tissues, with a failure to distinguish between "self" and "non-self". An immune response develops which may be specific for a particular organ, such as the thyroid gland, or react against a number of different organs, as in connective tissue diseases. The skin can manifest both types of autoimmune response. The results of such reactions can be destruction of the cells concerned and the production of inflammation. There is an inherited tendency to autoimmune disease, marked by specific HLA (human lymphocyte antigen) in some cases.

The most common types of skin disease in which this autoimmune mechanism occurs are the blistering disorders, pemphigoid and pemphigus, as well as dermatitis herpetiformis.

Direct immunofluorescence.

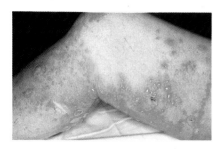

— Fluorescein labelled antibody to human immunoglobulin

— Antibody (immunoglobulin) in situ

— Normal antigen

— Skin section from patient

Indirect immunofluorescence.

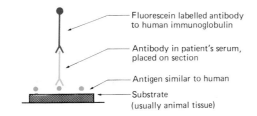

— Fluorescein labelled antibody to human immunoglobulin

— Antibody in patient's serum, placed on section

— Antigen similar to human

— Substrate (usually animal tissue)

Pemphigoid

This is a condition in which there are antibodies attached to the upper layer of the basement membrane at the dermo-epidermal junction with an underlying inflammatory reaction producing a split above the basement membrane. Lysosomal enzymes are released damaging the basement membrane, resulting in separation of the epidermis and blister formation. The presence of antibodies, usually IgG, can be demonstrated by an antihuman IgG antibody labelled with fluorescein. When viewed under the microscope with ultraviolet light illumination, the presence of the IgG antibody is shown by fluorescence. The presence of circulating antibasement membrane antibodies can be shown either by direct immunofluorescence using a specimen of the patient's skin or by incubation by attachment to skin which has been incubated in serum from the patient.

As described in the section on blistering diseases, pemphigoid is a condition in which large tense blisters develop, frequently with an erythematous background, on the limbs, trunk, and flexures. It is mainly seen in the elderly and is slightly more common in women.

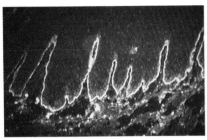

Indirect immunofluorescence.

Pemphigoid responds to treatment with prednisolone and, as might be expected, immunosuppressant drugs such as azathioprin. Another type of pemphigoid occurs in which there is scarring of the oral mucous membrane and the conjunctiva. Occasionally localised lesions are seen on the legs with evidence of an immune reaction, but often the absence of circulating antibasement membrane antibodies. This is a relatively benign condition and often responds to topical steroids.

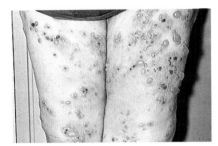

Pemphigus

In this condition, antibodies are found to have developed against the epidermis above the basement membrane. As a result of this reaction, there is separation of the epidermal cells with the formation of a superficial blister. Direct immunofluorescence of the skin from affected patients shows that antibodies are deposited on the intercellular substance of the epidermis. Oral lesions are much more common than in pemphigoid.

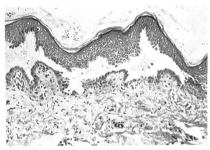

Intraepidermal split.

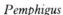

Direct immunofluorescence.

Pemphigus is a condition of middle age, although it is also seen in the elderly and blisters develop over the scalp, face, back, chest, and flexures. They also present as crusted erosions because the blister is so superficial that it readily breaks down. Rubbing the apparently unaffected skin may produce superficial erosions, the Nikolsky sign.

Pemphigus may also present with thickened hypertrophic lesions in pemphigus vegitans or with shallow erosions and scaling on the face and scalp in pemphigus foliaceous. It may be associated with myasthenia gravis in which there are antibody reaction to the cells of the thymus.

This condition requires more vigorous treatment than pemphigoid, usually with high doses of steroids and azathioprine.

Other organ-specific autoimmune diseases of the skin

Vitiligo—This is a condition where there is a loss of pigment as a result of antibodies developing against melanocytes in the skin in a limited area. However the areas affected tend to gradually increase. There may be other autoimmune diseases in the same patient, causing, for example, pernicious anaemia.

Alopecia areata—This condition may also be associated with an immune reaction against the hair follicle and, in addition, antibodies may develop to other organs such as the thyroid and gastric parietal cells.

Range of autoimmune disease

Organ specific   Hashimoto's thyroiditis
　　　　　　　　Pernicious anaemia
　　　　　　　　Addison's disease
　　　　　　　　Myasthenia gravis
　　　　　　　　Pemphigus
　　　　　　　　Pemphigoid
　　　　　　　　Primary biliary cirrhosis
　　　　　　　　Rheumatoid arthritis
　　　　　　　　Dermatomyositis
　　　　　　　　Systemic sclerosis
Non-organ specific   Lupus erythematosus

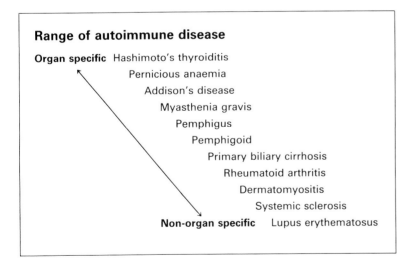

Clinical variants of lupus erythematosus

Systemic
Subacute cutaneous
Discoid
(Neonatal)

Non-organ-specific skin autoimmune disease

Systemic lupus erythematosus (SLE)—The hallmark of this condition is the presence of antibodies against various components of the cell nucleus. Although a wide range of organs may be affected, in three-quarters of the patients the skin is involved, generally with an erythematous eruption occurring bilaterally on the face in a "butterfly" distribution. There may also be photosensitivity, hair loss, and areas of vasculitis in the skin. There is frequently intolerance of sunlight. Subacute lupus erythematosus is a variant that presents with an erythematous eruption in the skin and anticytoplasmic RNA antibodies.

Immunology and the skin

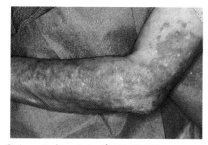

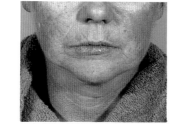

Subacute lupus erythematosus.

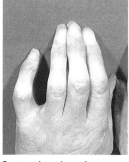

Discoid lupus erythematosus.

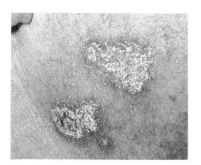

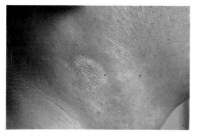

Systemic sclerosis. Morphoea.

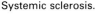

CREST syndrome

C—Calcinosis cutis
R—Raynaud's phenomenon
E—Esophagus
S—Scleroderma
T—Telangiectasia

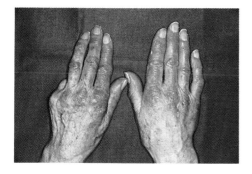

Discoid lupus erythematosis (DLE)—This is a condition in which circulating antinuclear antibodies are very rare. There are quite well defined inflammatory lesions, with some degree of atrophy occurring on the face and occasionally on the arms as well.

Treatment of SLE with the threatened or actual involvement of other organs is important. Prednisolone is usually required and sometimes immunosuppressant drugs such as azathioprine as well. Treatment of DLE is generally with topical steroids. Hydroxychloro- quine by mouth is also used, generally in a dose of 200 mg daily. This drug can diminish visual acuity and this should be checked every few months. A simple chart, the Amsler Chart, is available for patients to use, consisting of a central dot with a grid which becomes blurred when held at arm's length when there is any impairment of acutity.

Systemic sclerosis—This is a condition in which there is extensive sclerosis of the subcutaneous tissues in the fingers and toes as well as around the mouth (scleroderma), with similar changes affecting the internal organs, particularly the lung and kidneys. There are vascular changes producing Reynaud's phenomenon and telangiectasia around the mouth and on the fingers. It is associated with antinuclear antibodies (speckled or nucleolar), and in about 50% of cases, circulating immune complexes may be present. Endothelial cell damage in the capillaries results in fibrosis and sclerosis of the organs concerned. There is considerable tethering of the skin on the fingers and toes, which becomes very tight with a waxy appearance and considerable limitation of movement. A variant is the CREST syndrome.

Morphoea is a benign form of localised systemic sclerosis in which there is localised sclerosis with very slight inflammation. There is atrophy of the overlying epidermis. The early changes often consist of a dusky appearance to the skin.

Dermatomyositis—This condition is characterised by a red violet discoloration of the skin known as "heliotrope" on the back of the hands and over the eyelids. There may be involvement of the cheeks and forehead as well. The finding of muscle weakness together with specific electromyographic changes and an inflammatory infiltrate in the muscle means there is almost certainly an underlying malignancy, so suitable investigation is indicated. There are a number of cases in which removal of the offending neoplasm has resulted in resolution of the skin and muscle lesions.

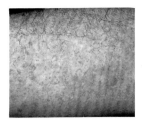

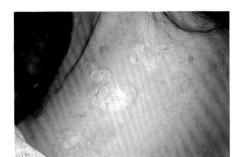

Lichen sclerosus—This is a relatively uncommon condition seen mainly in women in which well defined patches of superficial atrophy of the epidermis occur with a white colour. There is fibrosis of the underlying tissues. It frequently occurs in the vulva and perineum and may also appear on the penis as *balanitis xerotica obliterans*. Extragenital lesions may occur anywhere on the skin. It may occur in a more acute form in children where it tends to resolve, but in adults it is a very chronic condition. There is an increased incidence of squamous cell carcinoma. Treatment is with topical steroids and excision of any areas that appear to be developing tumours.

Graft versus host disease—This reaction occurs following bone marrow transplantation in immunosuppressed patients. T lymphocytes produced by the graft react against the body's own tissues, producing a skin eruption which may resemble measles. There is lysis of the basement membrane with shedding of the skin and sometimes lichen planus like eruption. In the more chronic form, localised lesions develop, with immunoglobulins deposited in the walls of blood vessels with the activation of complement.

Further reading

Roitt IM, Brostoff J, Male D. *Immunology*. 4th ed. St Louis: Mosby, 1995.

22. THE SKIN AND SYSTEMIC DISEASE

When a man has on the skin of his body a swelling or an eruption or a spot . . . and the disease appears to be deeper than the skin it is a leprous disease.

Leviticus 13:2-3

Although arguments continue about what the Old Testament writers understood by "leprous", there was clearly an appreciation of the connection between the skin and systemic illness. As in ancient times, clinical signs in the skin may give valuable diagnostic clues to underlying disease. Sometimes the same condition affects both the skin and other organs, or severe skin disease itself may be the cause of generalised illness.

The skin is also a common target organ for allergic reactions to drugs, with a rash being the first clinical sign. The florid skin lesions of AIDS illustrate the results of infections when the immune response is impaired.

The cutaneous signs of systemic disease is a very large subject, on which much has been written, so the presence of a skin eruption that might indicate systemic disease is good reason to consult the large textbooks. Nevertheless, it is possible to give an outline of the more common skin changes that may be associated with systemic illness.

Erythematous rashes

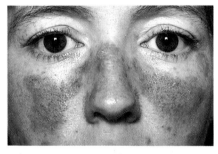

Systemic lupus erythematosus.

Lupus erythematosus—There are two forms of this condition: *discoid*, which is limited to the skin, and *systemic*, in which the skin changes are associated with disease of the kidneys and other organs. The acute, erythematous rash on the malar area of the face, usually in a woman, is characteristic of the systemic type. In discoid lupus erythematosus there are well defined lesions, which are a combination of atrophy and hyperkeratosis of the follicles, giving a "nutmeg grater" feel. It occurs predominantly on the face or areas exposed to the sun, as chronic, erythematous lesions that are much worse in the summer months.

Allergic reactions to drugs, commonly the penicillins—There may be a widespread rash developing from a few days to two weeks after treatment with moderate illness (type III) or an acute life threatening anaphylactic reaction (types I and III) with acute angio-oedema and renal failure. A fixed drug eruption is characterised by a localised patch of erythema that flares up whenever the drug is taken.

Infection—The characteristic rash of the various viral infections is, in a broad sense, also an allergic response. Less specific reactions such as erythema multiforme are commonly associated with infection—for example, herpes and other viral infections and streptococcal infection—but also with connective tissue disease and drugs such as sulphonamides.

In *carcinoid and phaeochromocytoma* vasoactive substances cause episodes of flushing and telangiectasia.

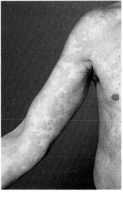

Rash from penicillin.

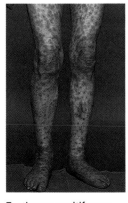

Erythema multiforme.

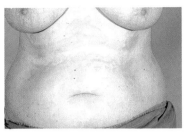

Figurate erythema.

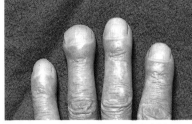

Erythema of nailbeds and clubbing.

Neoplasia—Numerous patterns of widespread erythema have been described—the *"figurate erythemas"*—which may be associated with underlying carcinoma. *Dermatomyositis*, also a rare condition, has very high association in adults with underlying carcinoma commonly of the breasts, lung, ovary, or gastrointestinal tract. It is characterised by localised erythema with a purple hue, predominantly on the eyelids, cheeks, and forehead. There may be similar changes on the dorsal surface of the fingers often with dilated nail fold capillaries. These changes may precede the discovery of an underlying tumour and may also fade away once it is removed. There is variable association with muscle aching and weakness.

Erythema of the nailbeds may be associated with connective tissue disease—such as lupus erythematosus, scleroderma, and dermatomyositis. "Clubbing" of the fingers may be associated.

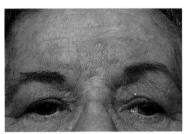

Dermatomyositis.

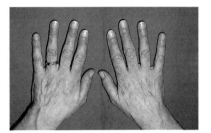

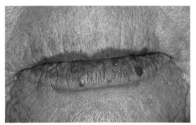

CREST syndrome.

Telangiectasia and clubbing may be features of scleroderma in the CREST syndrome. In this type of scleroderma there are **C**alcium deposits below the skin on the fingers and toes, **R**aynaud's phenomenon with poor peripheral circulation, immobility of the o**E**sophagus, dermal **S**clerosis of the fingers and toes, and **T**elangiectasia of the face and lips and adjacent to the toe and finger nails.

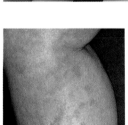

Erythrocyanosis is a dusky, red, cyanotic change in the skin over the legs and thighs, where there is a deep layer of underlying fat. The condition becomes worse in the winter months. It is most common in young women and usually resolves over the years. Lupus erythematosus, sarcoidosis, and tuberculous infection may localise in affected areas.

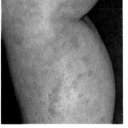

Livedo reticularis is a cyanotic, net-like discoloration of the skin over the legs. It may be idiopathic or associated with arteritis or changes in blood viscosity.

Spider naevi, which show a central blood vessel with radiating branches, are frequently seen in women (especially during pregnancy) and children. If they occur in large numbers, particularly in men, they may indicate liver failure. Palmar erythema and yellow nails may also be present.

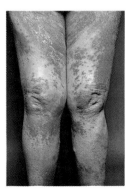

Vasculitis.

Vasculitis and purpura of the skin may be associated with disease of the kidneys and other organs, as has already been discussed. "Splinter haemorrhages" under the nails are usually the result of minor trauma but may be associated with a wide range of conditions, including subacute bacterial endocarditis and rheumatoid arthritis.

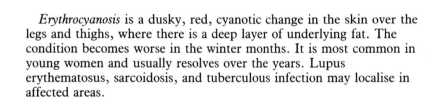

101

Changes in pigmentation

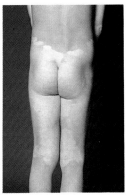

Vitiligo.

Hypopigmentation

A widespread partial loss of melanocyte functions wih loss of skin colour is seen in hypopituitarism and is caused by an absence of melanocyte stimulating hormone. In the various types of autosomal recessive albinism there is a very considerable loss of pigment from the skin, hair, and eyes.

Localised depigmentation is most commonly seen in vitiligo, in which a family history of the condition is found in one third of the patients. In the sharply demarcated, symmetrical macular lesions there is loss of melanocytes and melanin. There is an increased incidence of organ specific antibodies and their associated diseases.

Autoimmune associations with vitiligo

Thyroid disease	Myasthenia gravis
Pernicious anaemia	Alopecia areata
Hypoparathyroidism	Halo naevus
Addison's disease	Morphoea and
Diabetes	lichen sclerosus

Other causes of hypopigmented macules include: postinflammatory conditions following psoriasis, eczema, lichen planus, and lupus erythematosus; infections—for example, tinea versicolor and leprosy; chemicals, such as hydroquinones, hydroxychloroquine, and arsenicals; reactions to pigmented naevi, seen in halo naevus; and genetic diseases, such as tuberous sclerosis ("ash leaf" macules).

Hyperpigmentation

There is wide variation in the pattern of normal pigmentation as a result of heredity and exposure to the sun. Darkening of the skin may be due to an increase in the normal pigment melanin or to the deposition of bile salts in liver disease, iron salts (haemochromatosis), drugs, or metallic salts from ingestion.

Causes of hyperpigmentation include the following.

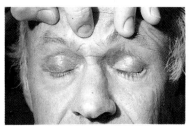

Argyria (silver salts in skin).

Hormonal—An increase in circulating hormones that have melanocyte stimulating activity occurs in hyperthyroidism, Addison's disease, and acromegaly. In women who are pregnant or taking oral contraceptives there may be an increase in melanocytic pigmentation of the face. This is known as melasma (or chloasma) and occurs mainly on the forehead and cheeks. It may fade slowly. Sometimes a premenstrual darkening of the face occurs.

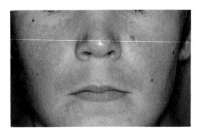

Melasma.

Increased deposition of haemosiderin is generalised in haemochromatosis. Localised red-brown discoloration of the legs is seen with longstanding varicose veins. It also occurs in a specific localised pattern in Schamberg's disease, when there is a "cayenne pepper" appearance of the legs and thighs.

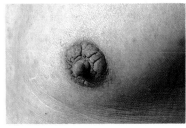

Acanthosis nigricans.

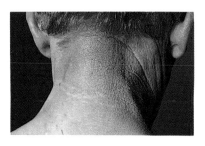

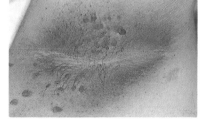

Pseudoacanthosis nigricans.

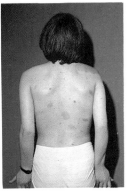
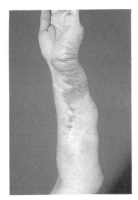

Neurofibromatosis.

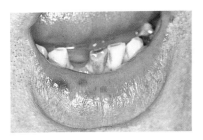

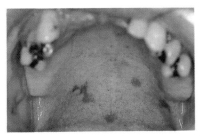

Peutz–Jeghers syndrome.

Neoplasia—Lymphomas may be associated with increased pigmentation. *Acanthosis nigricans*, characterised by darkening and thickening of the skin of the axillae, neck, nipples, and umbilicus, occurs with internal cancers, usually adenocarcinoma of the stomach. It is also seen in acromegally. There is a benign juvenile type. *Pseudoacanthosis nigricans* is much more common, consisting of simple darkening of the skin in the flexures of obese individuals; it is not associated with malignancy.

Drugs—Chlorpromazine, other phenothiazines, and minocycline may cause an increased pigmentation in areas exposed to the sun. Phenytoin can cause local hyperpigmentation of the face and neck.

Inflammatory reactions—Post inflammatory pigmentation is common, often following acute eczema, fixed drug eruptions, or lichen planus. Areas of lichenification from rubbing the skin are commonly darkened.

Malabsorption and deficiency states—In malabsorption syndromes, pellagra, and scurvy there is commonly increased skin pigmentation.

Congenital conditions—There is clearly a marked variation in pigmentation and in the number of freckles in normal individuals. There may be localised well defined pigmented areas in neurofibromatosis with "cafe au lait" patches. Increased pigmentation with a blue tinge occurs over the lumbosacral region in the condition known as Mongolian blue spot.

Peutz–Jeghers syndrome is inherited as an autosomal dominant characterised by pigmented macules of the oral mucosal membranes, lips, and face that appear in infancy. Benign intestinal polyps, mainly in the ileum and jejunum, which very rarely become malignant, are associated with the condition.

Malignant lesions

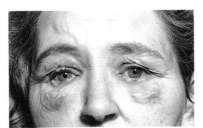

Lymphoma.

B cell lymphoma.

Malignant lesions may cause skin changes such as acanthosis nigricans and dermatomyositis or produce secondary lesions. Lymphomas can arise in or invade the skin and pruritus may be associated with Hodgkin's disease.

Mycosis fungoides is a T cell lymphoma of cutaneous origin. Initially well demarcated erythematous plaques develop on covered areas with intense itching. In many cases there is a gradual progression to infiltrated lesions, nodules, and ulceration. In others the tumour may occur de novo or be preceded by generalised erythema.

Skin markers of internal malignancy

- Acanthosis nigricans—usually intra-abdominal lesions
- Erythematous rashes, "figurate erythema"
- Pruritus—usually lymphoma
- Dermatomyositis in the middle aged and elderly
- Acquired ichthyosis

Poikiloderma, in which there is telangiectasia, reticulate pigmentation, atrophy, and loss of pigment, may precede mycosis fungoides, but it is also seen after radiotherapy and in connective tissue diseases.

Parapsoriasis is a term used for well defined maculopapular erythematous lesions that occur in middle and old age. Some cases undoubtedly develop into mycosis fungoides and a biopsy specimen should be taken of any such fixed plaques that do not clear with topical steroids.

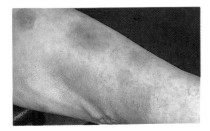

Parapsoriasis.

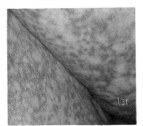

Poikiloderma.

The gut and the skin

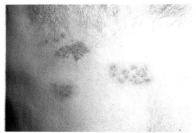
Early pyoderma gangrenosum.

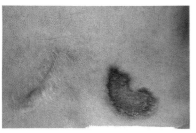
Pyoderma gangrenosum.

Pyoderma gangrenosum may occur with

- Ulcerative colitis
- Crohn's disease
- Rheumatoid arthritis
- Monoclonal gamopathy
- Leukaemia

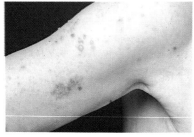
Dermatitis herpetiformis.

Liver disease and the skin

Obstructive:
  Jaundice
  Pruritus

Liver failure:
  Multiple spider naevi (in men)
  Palmar erythema
  White nails—hypoalbuminaemia
  Porphyria cutanea tarda

Cirrhosis:
  Xanthomas (primary biliary cirrhosis)
  Asteatosis

Vasculitis of various kinds, periarteritis nodosa, connective tissue diseases such as scleroderma, and many metabolic diseases produce both cutaneous and gastrointestinal lesions. There are, however, some specific associations.

Dry skin, asteatosis, and itching, with superficial eczematous changes and a "crazy paving" pattern, occur in malabsorption and cachectic states. Increased pigmentation, brittle hair and nails may also be associated.

Pyoderma gangrenosum—An area of non-specific inflammation and pustules breaks down to form a necrotic ulcer with hypertrophic margins. There is an underlying vasculitis. There is a strong association with ulcerative colitis and also with Crohn's disease, rheumatoid arthritis, abnormal gamma globulins and leukaemia.

Dermatitis herpetiformis, which has already been discussed, is an intensely itching, chronic disorder with erythematous and blistering lesions on the trunk and limbs. It is more common in men than women. Most patients have a gluten sensitive enteropathy with some degree of villus atrophy. There is an associated risk of small bowel lymphoma.

Other conditions—Peutz–Jeghers syndrome, with intestinal polyposis, has already been mentioned, but there are other rare congenital disorders with connective tissue and vascular abnormalities that affect the gut, such as Ehlers–Danlos syndrome and pseudoxanthoma elasticum (arterial gastrointestinal bleeding), purpuric vasculitis (bleeding from gastrointestinal lesions), and neurofibromatosis (intestinal neurofibromas).

Crohn's disease (regional ileitis)—Perianal lesions and sinus formation in the abdominal wall often occur. Glossitis and thickening of the lips and oral mucosa and vasculitis may be associated.

Liver diseases may affect the skin, hair and nails to a variable degree. Obstructive jaundice is often associated with a variable degree of itching which is thought to be due to the deposition of bile salts in the skin. Evidence of this is the fact that drugs which combine bile salts such as cholestyramine improve pruritus in some patients. Jaundice is the physical manifestation of bile salts in the skin.

Liver failure is characterised by a number of skin signs, particularly vascular changes causing multiple spider naevi and palmar erythema due to diffuse telangiectasia. It is not unusual to see spider naevi on the trunk in women but large numbers in men should raise suspicion of underlying hepatic disease.

Porphyria cutanea tarda as a result of chronic liver disease produces bullae, scarring and hyperpigmentation in sun-exposed areas of the skin. *Xanthomas* may be associated with primary biliary cirrhosis and in chronic liver disease asteotosis, with dry skin producing a crazy paving pattern',

Diabetes and the skin

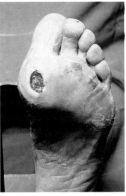
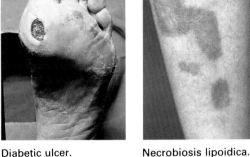

Diabetic ulcer.

Necrobiosis lipoidica.

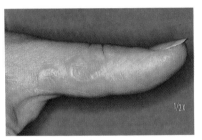

Granuloma annulare.

In diabetes the disturbances of carbohydrate-lipid metabolism, small blood vessel lesions, and neural involvement may be associated with skin lesions. The more common of these include the following.

Infection—Diabetic patients have an increased susceptibility to staphylococcal, coliform, and pseudomonal infection. *Candida albicans* infection is also more common in diabetics.

Vascular lesions—"Diabetic dermopathy," due to a microangiopathy, consists of erythematous papules which slowly resolve to leave a scaling macule on the limbs. Atherosclerosis with impaired peripheral circulation is often associated with diabetes.

Ulceration due to neuropathy (trophic ulcers) or impaired blood supply may occur, particularly on the feet.

Specific skin lesions

Necrobiosis lipoidica—40–60% of patients with this condition may develop diabetes but it is not very common in diabetic patients (0·3%). As the name indicates, there is necrosis of the connective tissue with lymphocytic and granulomatous infiltrate. There is replacement of degenerating collagen fibres with lipid material. It usually occurs over the shin but may appear at any site.

Granuloma annulare usually presents with localised papular lesions on the hands and feet but may occur elsewhere. The lesions may be partly or wholly annular and may be single or multiple. There is some degree of necrobiosis with histiocytes forming "palisades" as well as giant cells and lymphocytes. It is seen more commonly in women, usually those aged under 30. There is an association with insulin dependent diabetes. In itself it is a harmless and self limiting condition that slowly clears but may recur.

Other diseases

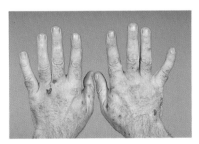
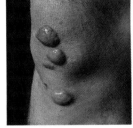

Porphyria.

Xanthomas.

Porphyrias are due to the accumulation of intermediate metabolites in the metabolic pathway of haem synthesis. There are several types. In hepatic porphyrias there is skin fragility leading to blisters from exposure to the sun or minor trauma. In erythropoietic and erythrohepatic photoporphyrias there is intense photosensitivity. They are sometimes associated with sensitivity to long wavelength ultraviolet light that penetrates window glass.

Porphyria cutanea tarda usually occurs in men, with a genetic predisposition, who have liver damage, as a result of an excessive intake of alcohol. There is impaired porphyria metabolism leading to skin fragility and photosensitivity, with blisters and erosions, photosensitivity on the face and the dorsal surface of the hands.

Xanthomas are due to the deposition of fat in connective tissue cells. They are commonly associated with hyperlipidaemia—either primary or secondary to diabetes, the nephrotic syndrome, hypothyroidism, or primary biliary cirrhosis. Four of the primary types are associated with an increased risk of atherosclerosis; type I is not. Diabetes may be associated with the eruptive type.

Necrotising fasciitis—An area of cellulitis that develops vesicles and necrosis of the skin may indicate much more extensive, life threatening necrosis of the deeper tissues. Urgent surgical debridement is indicated.

Amyloid deposits in the skin occur in primary systemic amyloidosis and myeloma.

Common types of xanthoma

Clinical type	Association with hyperlipidaemia	
	Primary type	Secondary
Xanthelasma of the eyelids—yellow plaques	II (may be normal)	–
Tuberous nodules on elbows and knees	II, III	+
Eruptive—small yellow papules on buttocks and shoulders	I, III, IV, V	+
Plane—yellow macules, palmar creases involved, generalised (myeloma)	I, III	+
Tendons—swelling on fingers or ankle	II, III	+

The skin and systemic disease

Pregnancy

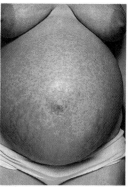

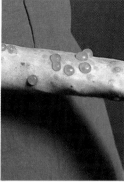

Polymorphic eruption.

Pemphigoid gestationis.

Pregnancy may be associated with pruritus, in which the skin appears normal in 15–20% of women (prunigo gestationis). It is generally more servere in the first trimester.

Polymorphic eruptions also present with pruritis with urticaria papules and plaques (the PUPP syndrome). It usually occurs on the abdomen in the third trimester and then becomes widespread. There may be a postpartrum flare up. It can be a distressing condition for the mother but the baby is not affected and it rarely recurs in subsequent pregnancies. Topical steroids can be used, but systemic steroids should be avoided.

Pemphigoid gestationis is a rare disorder that may resemble PUPP initially but develops pemphoid like vesicles, spreading over the abdomen and thighs: autoantibodies to the basement membrane are present.

Sarcoidosis

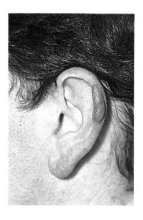

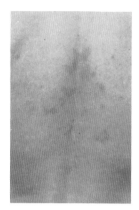

Sarcoidosis of the skin appears in various forms—as papules, nodules, plaques, or large cyanotic lesions ("lupus pernio"). Erythema nodosum may be associated.

Thyroid disease

Hypothyroidism	Hyperthyroidism
Dry skin	Soft, thickened skin
Oedema of eyelids and hands	Pretibial myxoedema
Absence of sweating	Increased sweating (palms and soles)
Coarse, thin hair—loss of pubic, axillary, and eyebrow hair	Thinning of scalp hair
Pale "ivory" skin	Diffuse pigmentation
Brittle poorly growing nails	Rapidly growing nails
Purpura, bruising, and telangiectasia	Palmar erythema
	Facial flushing

Thyroid disease is associated with changes in the skin, which may sometimes be the first clinical signs. There may be evidence of the effect of altered concentrations of thyroxine on the skin, with changes in texture and hair growth. Associated increases in thyroid stimulating hormone concentration may lead to pretibial myxoedema. In autoimmune thyroid disease vitiligo and other autoimmune conditions may be present.

Systemic malignancy

Skin signs of malignant disease

- Secondary deposits
- Secondary hormonal effects
  — Acne (adrenal tumours)
  — Flushing (carcinoid)
  — Pigmentation
- Generalised pruritus (particularly lymphoma)
- Figurate erythema
- Superficial thrombophlebitis
- Dermatomyositis
- Acanthosis nigricans
- Various eruptive skin lesions seen in Gardener's and Bazex syndromes

Genetics and skin disease

The fault, dear Brutus, is not in our stars but in ourselves
SHAKESPEARE, *Julius Caesar*, Act I Sc 2.

The knowledge that there may be underlying inherited factors when external causes have been excluded often helps patients come to terms with chronic skin disease that is otherwise inexplicable.

The commonest skin diseases, psoriasis and eczema, tend to run in families, suggesting that genetic factors are involved. Evidence for this in psoriasis is the association with the presence of antigens of the histocompatibility complex HLA-CW6. Recently HLA associated genes on chromosome 6 have been identified. The fact that when one parent is affected a child has a 25% chance of developing the disease suggests an autosomal dominant gene with partial penetrance. In atopic eczema the pattern of inheritance is not clearly defined and there is great variability in the degree to which associated conditions (asthma, hay fever, food allergies, and raised IgE levels) are present.

The HLA (histocompatibility antigens). These antigens occurring on the surface of cells play a critical role in the recognition by the body's immune system of tissues as belonging to the same individual. This distinction between 'self' and 'non self' is fundamental in matching organs from donor to recipient. The production of HLA antigens is controlled by a locus on the short arm of chromosome 6. So far five specific loci have been identitified, known as ABCD and DR. The presence of HLA antigens may be associated with a tendency to specific diseases such as psoriasis mentioned above, but also dermatitis herpetiformis, pemphigus, and Reiter's disease. It is possible that the development of autoimmune disease is associated with the development of antibodies to specific HLA antigens with a failure to recognise these as being 'self'.

Skin conditions with autosomal *dominant* inheritance include neurofibromatosis, acute intermittent porphyria, tuberous sclerosis, and the less severe forms of ichthyosis and epidermolysis bullosa.

Autosomal *recessive* inheritance is responsible for the more severe forms of ichthyosis and epidermolysis bullosa as well as other rare diseases such as xeroderma pigmentosa.

X linked genes are responsible for rare disorders such as incontinentia pigmenti in which epidermal growth is abnormal. Blistering, warty, and pigmented lesions occur in whorls over the skin surface. These follow the lines of Blaschko, indicating the existence of a population of cells with a different X chromosome to the majority—an example of mosaicism. Central nervous system and skeletal abnormalities may be associated.

Recent advances in genetics, particularly gene mapping, are rapidly enlarging our understanding of the genetic basis of numerous diseases. This section indicates areas of relevance to dermatology that you may wish to pursue in larger texts.

Further reading

Braverman IM. *Skin signs of systemic disease*. 2nd ed. Philadelphia: Sanders, 1981.
Callen JP. *Dermatological signs of internal disease*. 2nd ed. Philadelphia: Saunders, 1995.
Moss C, Savin J. *Dermatology and the new genetics*. Oxford: Blackwell Science, 1995.
Sharvill DE. *Skin signs of systemic disease*. London: Gower Medical, 1988.

23. ULTRAVIOLET RADIATION AND THE SKIN

R StC Barnetson

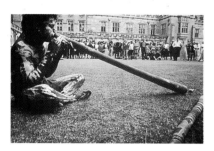

Aborigines do not get skin cancer

UVC	UVB*	UVA†	Visible	Infrared
Wavelength: (280 nm)	Short wave sunburn spectrum (280-320 nm)	Long wave (320-400 nm)	(380-770 nm)	(700 nm)‡

*The UVB band (280-320 nm) is responsible for erythema, sunburn, tanning and skin malignancy
†UVA light (320-400 nm) has the greatest penetration into the dermis and augments UVB erythema and perhaps skin malignancy.

Light spectrum

People with darkly pigmented skin very rarely get skin cancer. Those with fair skin, for example people of Celtic descent living in countries such as Australia, get skin cancer very readily. Australia has the highest incidence of skin cancer in the world, with 140,000 new cases per year, and 1200 deaths per year and 1200 deaths per year mainly from melanoma.

It is therefore important to understand that there is a variation in skin type, at present rated from 1 to 6 (Fitzpatrick classification). Skin type 1 subjects have red hair and do not tan, burn very easily in the sun and develop skin cancer very easily, whereas skin type 6 subjects have black skin (with an inbuilt sun protection factor of 10) and very rarely develop skin cancer.

Ultraviolet (UV) radiation is responsible for skin cancer; it is thought that visible light and infrared radiation are not important in carcinogenesis. UV radiation is split into three parts: UVC (200–290nm), UVB (290–320nm), and UVA (320–400 nm). UVC does not penetrate the stratosphere due to the ozone layer. UVB is very important in both sunburn and the development of skin cancer. UVA is thought to be of increasing importance in the development of skin cancer, and causes tanning but not sunburn. It is also important in people with photosensitivity. The effects of ultraviolet radiation may be classified as short term (sunburn, photosensitivity) or long term (skin cancer, wrinkling, solar elastosis, solar keratoses, seborrhoeic warts).

Photosensitivity is not uncommon, and is usually due to UVB or visible light. It is classified in the box below. The most common causes are drugs such as antibiotics, diuretics and psychotropics, and chemicals in industry.

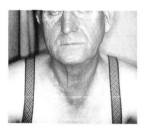

Photosensitivity caused by drugs

Skin types and sun

Type 1	Never tans, freckles, red hair, blue eyes
Type 2	Tans with difficulty, less freckled
Type 3	Tans easily, dark hair, brown eyes
Type 4	Always tans, Mediterranean skin
Type 5	Brown skin (e.g. Indian)
Type 6	Black skin (e.g. African)

Causes of photosensitivity

- Idiopathic, e.g. polymorphic light eruption, actinic prurigo, solar urticaria
- Photoaggravated dermatoses, e.g. lupus erythematosus, eczema
- Porphyria, e.g. erythropoietic, hepatic
- Drug induced, e.g. sulphonamides, phenothiazines
- Chemical induced (topical), e.g. tar, anthracene

Development of skin cancers

Sun-damaged skin
A number of different features characterise sun-damaged skin, which is often seen in the elderly particularly if they have lived in a sunny climate such as Australia. The skin has many fine wrinkles and often has a sallow yellowish discolouration particularly on the face and other exposed parts of the body. There may be hyperpigmentation, which may be diffuse as a result of recent sun exposure, or localised in the form of solar lentigo. In some areas there may be hypopigmentation, particularly where solar keratoses have been

Effects of sun

Short term
  1 Sunburn
  2 Photosensitivity

Long term
  1 Skin wrinkling
    Telangiectasia
    Hyper- and hypopigmentation
  2 Solar elastosis
  3 Actinic keratosis
    Seborrhoeic warts
  4 Skin cancers

treated with liquid nitrogen (cryotherapy). There may be marked telangiectasia and numerous blood vessels are seen. In some, there may be gross thickening of the skin particularly of the neck, due to elastin deposition in the upper dermis; this is known as solar elastosis.

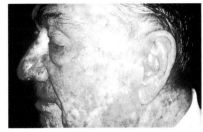

Sun damaged skin

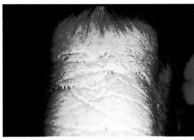

Solar elastosis

Dysplastic naevi

- Numerous moles
- Large moles, >1cm
- Irregular border, inflammatory flare
- Irregular pigmentation
- Histological "dysplasia"
- Familial tendency

Moles (melanocytic naevi)

These may be congenital (i.e. they are present at birth) or acquired. The latter are the more common, and are to some extent dependent on sunlight exposure, as children living in sunny places develop more than those in temperate climates. They may develop anytime in the first three decades of life.

Moles are a form of benign tumour, with a proliferation of melanocytes in the epidermis or dermis. The number of moles varies, but those with Type 1 or Type VI skin tend to have few, if any. In most, the melanocytes look relatively normal on histological examination, but in some there may be marked dysplasia (dysplastic naevi). In those with the dysplastic naevus syndrome, which in some patients is familial, there are many moles, which are irregular and large on clinical examination, and there may be more than a hundred in total. These people are liable to develop melanomas, and should be followed up on a routine basis, possibly with serial photographs.

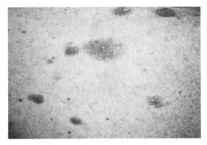

Dysplastic naevi

Premalignant tumours

There are three important forms of premalignant lesions: solar keratosis, Bowen's intraepidermal carcinoma leading to squamous cell carcinoma, and lentigo maligna leading to melanoma. Interestingly, basal cell carcinoma does not have a precursor. All these premalignant conditions may be present for several years before progressing on to the full-blown carcinoma.

Solar keratoses(SK) are scaly lesions which develop on sun-exposed sites, such as the face, the scalp in bald men, and the arms and legs. Some people have many SKs, particularly those with type 1 or type 2 skin. Most regress spontaneously in winter, but it is estimated that 1 : 1000 will progress on to squamous cell carcinoma (SCC). They are usually small, but may exceed 1cm in diameter with marked hyperkeratosis. If they become tender or painful, this suggests that they are progressing to SCC. The normal treatment of SKs is by curettage and cautery with liquid nitrogen (cryotherapy) or the topical application of an ointment 5-fluorouracil.

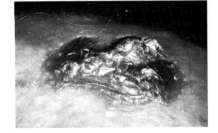

Solar keratoses

Bowen's intraepidermal carcinoma is a carcinoma in situ, with extension of the malignant keratinocytes in the epidermis in a phase of radial growth without invasion of the dermis. It presents clinically as a red plaque, which resembles psoriasis. It is painless, and may be present for many years before progressing to SCC, when a nodule develops within the plaque. The intraepidermal carcinoma is normally treated by cryotherapy, or possibly excision.

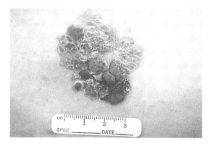

Bowen's intraepidermal carcinoma

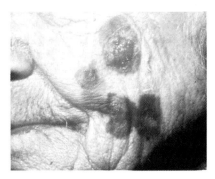

Lentigo maligna

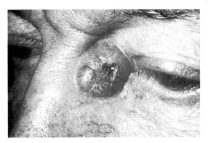

Basal cell carcinoma

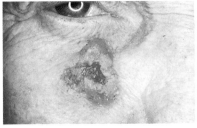

Squamous cell carcinoma

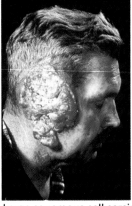

Large squamous cell carcinoma due to sun

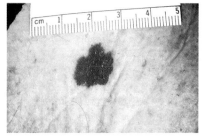

Superficial spreading malignant melanoma

Lentigo maligna is a lesion analogous to intraepidermal carcinoma. There are malignant melanocytes within the epidermis which extend radially with enlargement of the lentigo. Lentigo maligna may be present for many years (up to 20 years in some) before progressing to lentigo maligna melanoma. They are clinically characterised by the development of a black macule, usually on exposed sites such as the face, which grows very slowly.

Rising incidence of skin cancer

There are three common forms of skin cancer caused by ultraviolet light: basal cell carcinoma (BCC), squamous cell carcinoma (SCC), and malignant melanoma. Whereas there seems to be a direct relationship with the amount of UV exposure and BCC and SCC, the relationship with UV exposure and melanoma is more complex; it seems likely that intermittent exposure to UV light in melanoma is more important (e.g., exposure to sunlight on holidays).

BCC is by far the commonest of the skin cancers, and they occur de novo without a precursor lesion, usually on sun-damaged skin. They are thus common on the face and neck, particularly in the nodular form. They are characterised by their shiny, pearly nature; they often have blood vessels coursing over them and they may be ulcerated (hence the term rodent ulcer). When they occur on the trunk they tend to be macular, with areas of scarring due to spontaneous regression; these are known as superficial BCCs. BCCs very rarely metastasise, but are locally invasive, with the potential to destroy underlying structures such as bone. In some there is marked scar formation with spread around the nerves, so called morphoeic or cicatricial BCCs.

SCCs are less common than BCCs and they may metastasise and therefore kill the patient. They often develop from precursor lesions, such as solar keratoses and Bowen's intraepidermal carcinoma. Alternatively they can complicate chronic granulomatous conditions such as leprosy ulcers and skin tuberculosis. SCC usually presents as a ragged nodule or ulcer, which enlarges either slowly or rapidly. There may be associated lymphadenopathy, and metastasis to distant organs such as liver, lung and brain may occur. The diagnosis is made by performing a biopsy. Treatment modalities include excision, curettage, and cautery and radiotherapy.

Malignant melanoma is the most feared of the common skin tumours because it tends to metastasise early. It is usually a black tumour (*melanos* = black in Greek), though some lack pigment, so called amelanotic melanomas. They often develop from moles, but paradoxically are also common in people with type 1 skin, who often have few moles. People with atypical moles (dysplastic naevi) where the moles are numerous (more than 100 in total), large and irregular, are particularly prone to developing melanoma, and this tendency tends to run in families (familial melanoma).

Melanomas are usually related to sunlight exposure, which is characteristically intermittent. It is likely that people who are constantly exposed to the sun develop defensive mechanisms against melanoma development, such as thickening of the horny layer and epidermis; those who have intermittent UV exposure do not have such a defence mechanism. Some melanomas do not seem to be related to sun exposure, such as those occurring on the feet, acral lentiginous melanomas, and those in the mucous membranes, under the nails and on the genitals. However, the commonest types of melanoma, superficial spreading and nodular, do have a significant association with sun exposure; this is also true of lentigo maligna melanomas which develop following a usually long history of lentigo maligna

Melanomas are characteristically black, and they usually grow quickly. They may spread laterally initially (radial growth phase) and then become nodular (vertical growth phase). They may grow to a

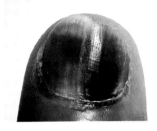

Subungual melamona

considerable size, being 3–4cm in diameter. The diagnosis is made by histological examination, preferably following excision of the tumour. The prognosis in the patient depends on the thickness of the tumour on histological examination, the Breslow thickness. If the tumour is less than 0.75mm then the chance of metastasis is 10%, if it is >3mm in thickness, then the chance of metastasis is more than 50%. Metastasis may occur within the skin, to the lymph nodes, or to distant organs such as liver, lung, and brain. When spread occurs to distant organs, death will almost certainly ensue. Spread to lymph nodes can now be diagnosed very accurately by using lymphoscintigraphy, where a dye is injected into the tumour site, and the draining lymph nodes are ascertained by following the path of the dye.

Treatment is by wide excision of the tumour to ensure that abnormal melanocytes at the periphery of the tumour have been removed. In thicker tumours, lymphoscintigraphy is mandatory, and the relevant lymph nodes should be examined and removed. If spread has occurred beyond the lymph nodes, then treatment can only be palliative, although on occasion secondary metastases have been excised successfully. Treatment options include chemotherapy, interferon \alpha , radiotherapy, and intra-arterial limb perfusion using chemotherapeutic agents such as melphalan.

Prevention of sun damage and skin cancer

It is obvious that prevention of sun damage and skin cancer will depend on reducing exposure to UV radiation. This can be achieved in a number of ways:

(1) Staying inside or under cover around the middle of the day: "Between eleven and three, stay under a tree" in the summer months.

(2) Covering the skin with clothes. It must be remembered however that light clothes such as shirts or blouses may only have a sun protection factor (SPF) of 4. A wide-brimmed hat is essential to protect the face and neck.

(3) Sunscreens will greatly reduce sun exposure for exposed parts such as the face and hands. Sunscreens are much more efficient than previously, particularly those with SPF > 30; they are now water resistant, and most have a broad spectrum, protecting against UVB and UVA. This is important because there is now increasing evidence that UVA is important in the development of skin cancer.

24. TROPICAL SKIN DISEASES

R StC Barnetson

Skin diseases in the tropics are extremely common, they are usually due to infections or infestations.

Bacterial infections

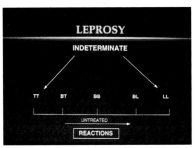

Leprosy spectrum TT = tuberculoid; BT = borderline tuberculoid; BB = borderline; BL = borderline lepromatous; LL = lepromatous leprosy

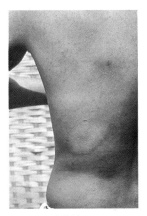

A tuberculoid leprosy

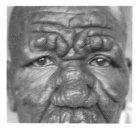

Lepromatous leprosy

Lepromatous leprosy: histology

Leprosy

This is still an important disease in the world; it maims rather than kills, and it causes major deformity in some due to nerve involvement. However, from a clinical point of view, it is mainly a skin disease. There are now about one million people with active disease in the world, 60% being in India.

The causative organism is *Mycobacterium leprae* which has a number of special characteristics:

(1) It is an obligate intracellular organism found in the skin, predominantly in macrophages, and in peripheral and dermal nerves within Schwann cells.

(2) It has a longer generation time than any other bacterium, which leads to a very long incubation period.

(3) It is an organism with a remarkable lack of toxicity; most manifestations of the disease are a result of the host response.

(4) It is highly infectious, contrary to popular belief; most contacts develop a subclinical infection, as is the case in tuberculosis.

Leprosy spectrum—There is a spectrum, both clinically and histologically, dependent on the immune response to the organism. Those with tuberculoid leprosy have a marked immune response to the bacterium, those with lepromatous leprosy do not. In between these two extremes, there lies borderline leprosy, with a spectrum comprising borderline tuberculoid, borderline and borderline lepromatous as the immune response diminishes.

Tuberculoid leprosy is characterised by localisation of the disease. Patients present with anaesthetic, anhidrotic, hypopigmented areas in the skin in darkly pigmented races; in South East Asians the areas are erythematous, dry, and anaesthetic. In lepromatous leprosy the disease is generalised, with characteristic nodular thickenings on the face and extremities. Nodules may also be found in the mouth, nose, and larynx; there may also be diffuse hypopigmentation. On histological examination, many viable bacilli are seen within the macrophages.

In borderline leprosy, a mixture of these two extreme pictures are seen. In borderline tuberculoid (BT) leprosy, there are widespread hypopigmented patches, and those with untreated BT leprosy generally tend to progress to the lepromatous end of the spectrum. In borderline lepromatous leprosy, the picture is similar to borderline tuberculoid leprosy, but the hypopigmented patches are less well demarcated, and bacilli are seen on histological examination. Borderline (BB) leprosy at the centre of the spectrum is an unstable state, with inflammation of the skin lesions halfway into reaction. A characteristic of this type of leprosy is the "ring lesion" where there is an area of normal skin within the inflamed area.

Reactions in leprosy—It is known that leprosy patients have acute episodes of inflammation, which are now recognised as being immunological reactions induced by hypersensitivity-type immunological reaction to bacillary antigens. Two types of reaction present commonly:

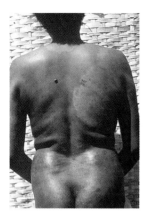
Borderline tuberculoid leprosy

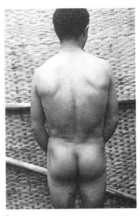
Borderline lepromatous leprosy

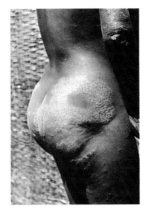
Borderline leprosy

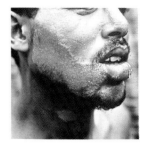
Borderline reactive leprosy

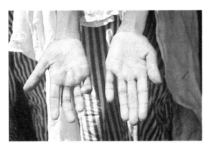
Ulnar deformity in leprosy

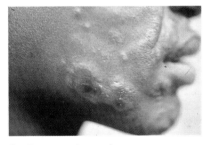
Erythema nodosum leprosum

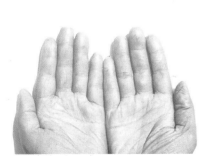
Dactylitis in erythema nodosum leprosum

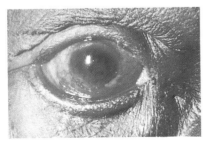
Iridocyclitis in erythema nodosum leprosum

Borderline leprosy reactions ("reversal reactions") present characteristically with swelling and erythema of previously hypopigmented skin lesions and the appearance of new lesions, and on occasion with severe oedema of the face and limbs. A marked feature of this type of reaction is neuritis with swelling and tenderness of the peripheral nerves. The neuritis may sometimes be the only presenting feature with no alteration in the skin lesions. If this neuritis is untreated, then permanent nerve damage due to granuloma formation and consequent scarring deformity is likely to result—neuritis in borderline leprosy reactions is the most important complication of the disease. Histologically, there is an increase in epithelioid cell granuloma formation in both skin and nerve, and in skin there is a tendency to develop more tuberculoid features. (Thus the term "reversal reaction", as there is an apparent reversal of the tendency of untreated borderline leprosy to become more lepromatous.) Immunological studies have shown that they are due to increased hypersensitivity to M. leprae, probably as a result of recognition of bacillary antigens in Schwann cells of peripheral and dermal nerves, where they have been sequestered undetected by the immune response. The exact triggers are unknown, but include viral infections, and parturition in pregnant mothers.

Borderline leprosy reactions may occur in both treated and untreated patients. With modern short courses of antileprosy drugs, these reactions frequently occur after the treatment is finished. It is important to treat the reactions early with oral corticosteroids before permanent nerve damage and deformity results.

Erythema nodosum leprosum (ENL) occurs only in patients with lepromatous and borderline lepromatous leprosy who develop tender erythmatous swollen skin lesions which tend to be smaller than those on borderline leprosy reactions, and more transient. Common concomitant manifestations are fever, neuralgia, and arthralgia. Less commonly, they may also have severe continuous neuritis, arthritis, dactylitis, orchitis, iridocyclitis and features of glomerulonephritis, with a clinical picture suggestive of serum sickness. The histology is typical of lepromatous leprosy, with the addition of foci of polymorphonuclear leucocytes, and evidence of vasculitis in some cases. The present evidence suggests that ENL is due to extravascular complex formation.

Episodes of ENL usually last a few days, and are often recurrent, particularly if there is concomitant infection with tuberculosis. On occasion ENL may lead onto borderline leprosy reactions. These reactions usually occur during treatment of the disease, but may occur after treatment when multidrug therapy is finished.

ENL is treated in the short term with non-steroidal anti-inflammatory drugs, or steroids, but if recurrent, it responds well to thalidomide. Episodes may be prevented by clofazimine, which is used as part of multidrug therapy.

Diagnosis of leprosy—The disease is best diagnosed by performing a skin biopsy. Skin smears from skin lesions are useful in multibacillary leprosy, particularly as a prognostic tool.

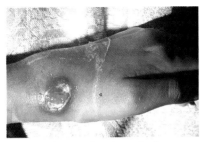

Primary chancre in tuberculosis

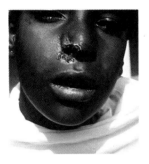

Lupus vulgaris in tuberculosis

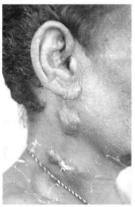

Scrofuloderma in tuberculosis

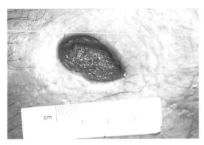

Buruli ulcer

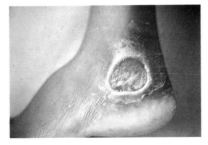

Tropical ulcer

Treatment of leprosy—

(1) Paucibacillary leprosy (TT, BT). Treatment is for 6 months, with dapsone 100mg daily, and rifampicin 600mg monthly.

(2) Multibacillary leprosy (BB, BL/LL). Treatment is with dapsone 100mg daily, clofazamine 300mg daily, and rifampicin 600mg per month. This treatment is continued for 2 years, or more if the skin smears remain positive for acid-fast bacilli.

Tuberculosis of the skin

Most cases of tuberculosis of the skin occur in the tropics where pulmonary tuberculosis is a common problem. Both human and bovine forms are implicated.

Primary tuberculosis skin infections usually occur in children. They result from trauma to the skin with introduction of the mycobacterial infection. A nodule develops usually on a limb, and becomes ulcerated. Secondary lesions then develop more proximally in a sporotrichoid fashion. Painless lymphadenitis may develop, and the lymph nodes may suppurate giving the clinical picture of scrofuloderma. The diagnosis is made by examination of pus from the primary ulcer which will reveal acid-fast bacilli.

Secondary tuberculosis skin infections may take a number of different forms, these include: lupus vulgaris, scrofuloderma, and verrucous tuberculosis.

Lupus vulgaris has a prolonged course and may have been present for 30 years or more. In light-skinned patients it has a characteristic brown colour, and diascopy reveals apple jelly nodules. Some plaques may become ulcerated leading eventually to marked disfigurement. It may affect the mucocutaneous functions, e.g. the nose.

Scrofuloderma is a very common form of secondary skin tuberculosis. It usually starts from a tuberculous focus in lymph nodes which then form sinuses in the skin. These are most commonly found on the neck and in the groin. They usually heal with marked scarring.

Verrucous tuberculosis commonly occurs on the buttocks and may result from intestinal tuberculosis. It may also occur in paramedical staff where it tends to occur on the arms and backs of hands from exposure to mycobacterial infection during autopsies.

The treatment of cutaneous tuberculosis is along established lines for pulmonary tuberculosis. Usually the treatment is with rifampicin, isoniazid, and ethambutol. Treatment should be continued until the lesions heal. Usually 6 months' treatment is adequate.

Buruli ulcer

This is due to *Mycobacterium ulcerans*, and most cases have been reported from Africa and Central America. Buruli ulcer is a chronic disease which starts 7–14 days after trauma to the affected area. The skin becomes red and oedematous with purple areas which become eschars. Ulcers develop with a formation of satellite ulcers interconnected by tunnels. These may extend along the limb, and surround it completely. This process may continue for several years. Diagnosis is made by examination of the necrotic tissue for acid-fast bacilli, and the organism can be cultured. Treatment depends on wide excision and debridement of the infected area, together with rifampicin and clofazimine given orally.

Tropical (phagedenic) ulcer

This is a common tropical condition. It is almost certainly an infective process, and recent research suggests that it may be due to a species of Fusobacterium. The organism is introduced into the skin through lacerations, and hence the ulcers are most common on the feet and lower legs. They usually present as a single ulcer which enlarges quickly, and may reach a diameter of 10 cm. It may be painful, and the borders are usually well defined. There is usually no fever or constitutional symptoms. The ulcer may heal after a week or two, or may progress to a chronic stage lasting for several years. Treatment is with intramuscular penicillin.

Fungal infections

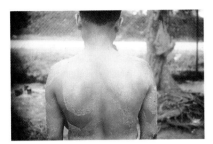

Tinea imbricata

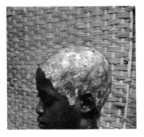

Favus

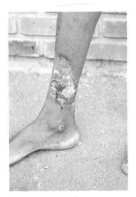

Sporotrichosis

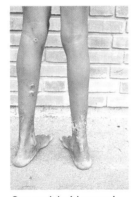

Sporotrichoid spread

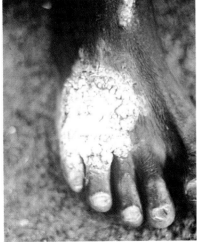

Chromomycosis

Superficial fungal infections

These infections, which are caused by the dermatophytes *Trichophyton*, *Epidermophyton* and *Microsporum*, are extremely common worldwide. They are also common in the tropics, and may be spread from human to human or from animal to human. Two varieties of superficial fungal infections are worthy of mention in the tropical context.

Tinea imbricata—This is common in South East Asia and the South Pacific, and is caused by Trichophyton concentricum. It starts as small light-brown papulovesicles which extend centrifugally to produce rosettes of concentric scaly rings. When these coalesce, they may cover large areas of the skin. As many exposed individuals remain unaffected, there may be a genetic factor which influences susceptibility. If infections are widespread, treatment with griseofulvin or other oral antifungal agents is indicated.

Favus—This is a form of scalp ringworm which has a very characteristic appearance. It is common around the Mediterranean, in the Middle East and in Asia. It is caused by *Trichophyton schoenleinii*. The patient is usually a child who develops diffuse widespread scaling of the scalp with characteristic shield-like scales. These are usually accompanied by a mousy odour. It is a chronic condition, which will progress to involve the whole scalp if adequate treatment is not instituted. The most effective treatment is griseofulvin which should be continued for 6 weeks.

Deep fungal infections

There are a large number of deep fungal infections, but three are worthy of mention as they occur worldwide, although most cases originate in tropical and subtropical regions with a hot humid climate.

Sporotrichosis—This is caused by the fungus *Sporothrix schenckii*. The fungus enters through a site of trauma to the skin and is thus commonly seen on the lower limbs. The incubation period is about 10 days.

The primary lesion is an ulcerated nodule or plaque which spreads in a very characteristic way along the lymphatic channels with skip lesions up the limbs ("sporotrichoid spread"). The nodules or plaques may persist for many years. Diagnosis is made by culture of the organism, as a skin biopsy may be unhelpful. The most effective treatment for sporotrichosis is potassium iodide in a saturated solution given orally over a period of 6–8 weeks. Itraconazole may also be effective.

Chromomycosis—This condition is common in Central and South America, Africa, the Far East, and the Western Pacific. It is caused by a number of fungi including *Phialophora, Fonsecaea, Cladosporium*, and *Rhinocladiella*. These organisms usually penetrate the skin via a trauma site, and are thus common on the foot and lower leg. Most patients are adult men.

The inoculation period is about 6 weeks. The characteristic lesion is a verrucous plaque which expands in size, but may spread in a way similar to sporotrichosis (sporotrichoid spread). The diagnosis is made when a biopsy of a plaque shows brown, thick-walled fungal cells with occasional hyphae. The treatment depends somewhat on the causative organism. In general, the current drug of choice is itraconazole which should be continued for 6 months, or until the plaque disappears.

Mycetoma (madura foot)—This is a subcutaneous infection caused either by actinomycetes (e.g. *Streptomyces, Nocardia*) or true fungi (e.g. *Madurella, Fusarium*, or *Aspergillus*). It is common in certain

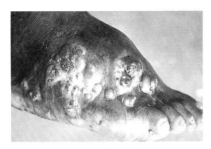

Myecetoma

Protozoan infestations

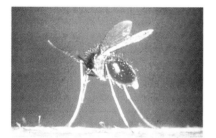

Sandfly, vector for leishmaniasis

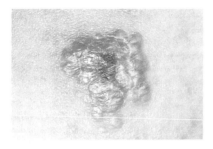

"Oriental sore" in leishmaniasis

parts of the tropics and subtropics, often in areas where there is a low annual rainfall. The main regions for the infections are Africa, the Middle East, India, and Central and South America. It is commoner in males than females, particularly occurring in agricultural workers who develop the infection following a penetrating injury to the foot, leg, or hand.

The first sign of mycetoma is the development of symptomless dermal or subcutaneous swelling, usually on the foot. In due course this swelling enlarges, and sinuses appear which extrude coloured material. There may be considerable woody swelling at this stage, accompanied by deformity. The main areas affected are the limbs, but it may occur on the trunk due to infection with Nocardia. Some infections may be extensive, but wide dissemination is rare. Osteomyelitis occurs commonly, as can be shown on X-ray.

The diagnosis is made by the demonstration of coloured grains containing the organism, obtained by opening a sinus. These can be observed by direct microscopy, and can be cultured to confirm the organism involved, which is important as the treatment of mycetoma depends on the organisms involved. Infections caused by actinomycetes can be treated with sulphonamides, rifampicin, and streptomycin. The treatment of fungal mycetoma (eumycetomas) is more difficult, but ketoconazole and itraconazole may be effective. In severe cases amputation of the foot may be indicated.

Cutaneous leishaniasis
This is a common skin disease in the Middle East, North Africa, and the Horn of Africa (Old World leishmaniasis), and Central and South America (New World leishmaniasis).

Old World leishmaniasis is a zoonosis which is spread to humans by sandflies; the primary host is usually a rat, gerbil, hyrax, (a rodent) or dog. The organisms responsible are the protozoa *Leishmania tropica*, *L major*, and *L aethiopica*. The clinical picture caused depends to some extent on the type of protozoa involved, *L tropica* and *L major* cause chronic boil-like nodules, usually on exposed skin, which may ulcerate (oriental sore) and in due course resolve spontaneously, usually within a year. Lesions are usually single, but in non-immune subjects may be multiple, even up to a hundred lesions. In a small number of cases, however, the disease may become progressive and may last for several years, with an expanding edge and central scarring; this is particularly common on the face. This is known as leishmaniasis recidivans, or lupoid leishmaniasis (resembling lupus vulgaris). Infections with *L major* may spread in the lymphatics (sporotrichoid spread), which gives a characteristic appearance. In *L aethopica* infections the skin lesions are more chronic, mucocutaneous involvement is common, and some patients develop widespread infections resembling lepromatous leprosy, diffuse cutaneous leishmaniasis.

The diagnosis may be made by taking a biopsy from the nodule, and demonstrating leishmania amastigotes within the macrophages of the dermal infiltrate, or in the serous fluid. Cautery or cryotherapy may be used to treat small lesions; another useful topical treatment is aminosidine ointment but this needs to be applied to the oriental sore for 12 weeks. Antimonial drugs given intralesionally or intramuscularly are also effective, and will be necessary for more severe infections.

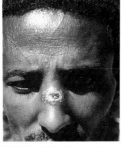

Old World leishmaniasis

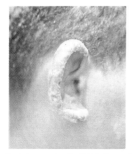

Leishmaniasis "chicleros"

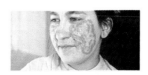

Leishmaniasis recidivans

New World leishmaniasis often presents a different clinical picture, the causative organisms are *L braziliensis* and *L mexicana*; the primary host is usually a forest rodent such as rice-rats and marmosets. A number of clinical forms are recognised including the chiclero's ulcer on the pinna of the ear espundia, with mucocutaneous involvement of the nose and mouth from secondary spread, and diffuse cutaneous leishmaniasis. Treatment is with sodium stibogluconate, meglumine antimonate, or ketaconazole.

Helminth infestations

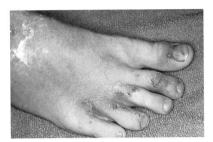

Cutaneous larva migrans

Cutaneous larva migrans (creeping eruption)
This is a relatively common condition in Asia, Africa, and Central America. It usually results from infestation with the larva of a dog or cat hookworm, for example, *Ancylostoma caninum*. It is commonly contracted on the beach by skin contact with dog faeces which contain the larvae, and for this reason it is common on feet, legs, and buttocks.

It presents as a linear urticarial intensely itching lesion which progresses a few centimetres each day due to the larvae moving within the skin. Eventually the larvae die, and the condition resolves spontaneously. The best treatment is 10% thiabendazole ointment topically.

Onchocerciasis
This is a disease of skin and other tissues and is a major cause of blindness (river valley blindness). It is caused by a filarial worm, Onchocerca volvulus. Adult worms, which are the thickness of a hair, are about 30 cm long and are found in the subcutaneous tissues where they may form fibrous nodules. The females produce microfilariae which invade the skin and eyes. The vector of the disease is a blackfly of the family Simuliidae, one important example in Africa being *Simulium damniosum*. It is estimated that there are about fifteen million patients in the world. It is common in tropical Africa, and Central and South America.

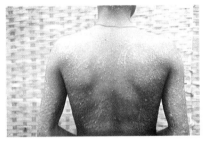

Onchocerciasis with marked lichenification

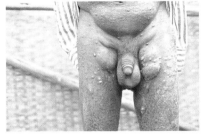

"Hanging groins" in onchocerciasis

Clinical manifestations—Repeated infestations are necessary to produce the full-blown disease. Often it presents with a chronic, itchy dermatitis, which is often localised to one limb ("unilateral scabies"); this progresses to a widespread dermatitis, with marked lichenification. In later stages the skin becomes "lizard-like" and the patient may develop "hanging groins". Inguinal lymphadenopathy is common, as are fibrous nodules in the skin containing the adult worms. Ultimately depigmentation may occur. The eyes are frequently invaded by microfilariae, which can be seen with a slit lamp in the anterior chamber of the eye, or in the cornea with intense infestations—blindness will result.

The diagnosis is made by taking a skin snip. A small needle is inserted into the skin, and the skin surrounding the needle is removed with a scalpel blade. This is placed on a slide in saline, and in about 30 minutes microfilaria will be seen under the microscope. The most effective treatment of onchocerciasis is with ivermectin, which kills the microfilariae.

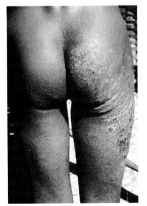

"Unilateral scabies" in onchocerciasis

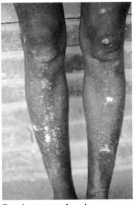

Depigmentation in onchocerciasis

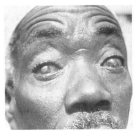

Blindness in onchocerciasis

FORMULARY

A great variety of preparations is available for treatment of skin conditions, and this list is limited to those in common use. There are numerous effective alternatives and it is inevitable that some medications have been omitted.

Topical treatment

General

The epidermis is capable of absorbing both greasy and aqueous preparations or a mixture of the two. The following should be used:

- Greasy ointments for dry scaling skin
- Watery creams for crusted weeping lesions
- Pastes where long action or occlusion is needed
- Gels for the face and scalp

Composition of bases

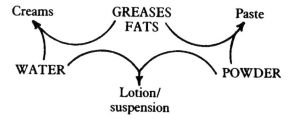

The consistency and properties of ointment and cream depend on the ratio of oil or grease to water (that is, whether they are oil in water or water in oil) and the emulsifying agents used—for example, emulsifying ointment contains soft white paraffin, emulsifying ointment and liquid paraffin.

The oils and greases range from mineral oil through soft paraffin to solid waxes. Some are naturally occurring, such as lanolin and beeswax. Creams or ointments may be used on their own as emollients or as vehicles for active ingredients.

Emollients—official preparations

Soft white paraffin—Greasy; protects skin and is long lasting.

Emulsifying ointment—Less greasy; mixes with water and can be used for washing.

Aqueous cream—Oil in water emulsion; useful as a vehicle, as an emollient, and for washing.

Liquid paraffin/white soft paraffin, equal parts—Spreads easily and is less greasy than white soft paraffin.

Hydrophilic ointment—Contains propylene glycol; mixes with water and spreads easily.

Lanolin (hydrous wool fat)—The natural emollient from sheep; mixes with water and greases, softens the epidermis, but can also cause allergic reactions.

Proprietary preparations

Proprietary preparations are numerous, varied, and more expensive than the standard preparations. They may also contain sensitisers—lanolin and preservatives (hydroxybenzoate, chlorocresol, sorbic acid)—and can cause allergies. Some examples are E45 cream (Crookes), Oilatum cream (Stiefel), and Lacticare (Stiefel), Unguentum Merck (Merck), Aquadrate (Norwich Eaton), and Diprobase (Schering-Plough).

Bath additives

Bath additives comprise dispersible oils such as Oilatum (Westwood, United States), Aveeno (Bioglan), Balneum (Merck), Alpha Keri, Westwood, United States), Emulsiderm (Dermal).

Treatment for psoriasis

Tar preparations—Various vehicles are used, generally pastes as these remain on the skin longer and have a prolonged effect. In treatment centres the standard coal tar preparations can be used, but these are difficult to use at home. Coal tar paste contains a strong solution of coal tar of 7·5% in 25 g of zinc oxide, 25 g of starch, and 50 g of white soft paraffin.

In Edinburgh hospitals 0·5%–4% crude coal is used with 15% zinc oxide in yellow soft paraffin. It is easy to use and effective but has a strong, distinctive smell. A more pleasant mixture is 10% strong coal tar solution and 2% salicylic acid in Unguentum Merck. The salicylic acid helps to soften thick keratotic scales.

There are numerous proprietary preparations that are less messy and do not stain but are not so effective. They are useful for treating less severe psoriasis at home. Examples are: Alphosyl cream (Stafford-Miller), Pragmatar (Bioglan), Psoriderm (Dermal). Alphosyl HC (Stafford-Miller) and Carbo-Cort (Lagap) contain hydrocortisone as well.

Ichthammol is a useful soothing extract of shale tar. It can be made up as a 1% paste in yellow soft paraffin with 15% zinc oxide.

Bath preparations—Bath preparations are useful for widespread psoriasis. Coal tar solution (20%) can be used or Polytar Emollient (Stiefel) or Psoriderm.

Tar shampoos are useful for treating psoriasis of the scalp. Polytar (Stiefel), T-Gel (Neutrogena), Capasal (Dermal), and Alphosyl (Stafford-Miller) are some examples.

Dithranol—Dithranol can be used in a paste containing salicylic acid, zinc oxide, starch, and soft white paraffin. It has to be applied carefully as it can cause severe irritation, avoiding contact with the surrounding skin.

For short contact treatment relatively clean preparations in a range of concentrations are available, such as Dithrocream (Dermal), Anthranol (Stiefel), and Psoradrate cream (Stafford-Miller).

Topical steroids

Topical steroids provide effective anti-inflammatory treatment but have the disadvantage of causing atrophy (due to decreased fibrin formation) and telangiectasis. They are readily absorbed by thin skin around the eyes and in flexures. On the face the halogenated steroids produce considerable telangiectasia so nothing stronger than hydrocortisone should be used (except in lupus erythematosus). They can cause hirsutism and folliculitis or acne. Infection of the skin may be concealed (Tinea incognita, for example) or made worse.

Side effects can be avoided by observing the following guidelines:
* Avoid long term use of strong steroids
* Potent or very potent steroids should be applied sparingly and often for a short time, then a less potent preparation less often as the condition improves
* Use only mildly potent steroids (that is, hydrocortisone) on the face
* Use preparations combined with antibiotics or antifungals for the flexures.

Topical steroids come in various strengths and a wide variety of bases—ointments, creams, oily creams, lotions, and gels—which can be used according to the type of lesion being treated.

Their pharmacological activity varies and they are classified according to their potency, the synthetic halogenated steroids being much stronger than hydrocortisone.

* Mildly potent   —Hydrocortisone 0·5, 1, and 2·5%
* Moderately potent—Eumovate (Glaxo), Stiedex LP (Stiefel);
* Potent   —Betnovate (Glaxo); Cutivate (Glaxo); Locoid (Brocades); and Synalar (Zeneca)
* Very potent   —Dermovate (Glaxo).

In Britain a full list showing relative potencies appears in *MIMS*.

Combinations with antiseptics and antifungals.

* Mildly potent   —Vioform HC (Zyma)
  —Terra-Cortril ointment (Pfizer), containing oxytetracycline and hydrocortisone
  —Fucidin H cream or ointment (Leo) containing fucidic acid and hydrocortisone
  —Canesten HC (Baypharm)
  —Daktacort cream (Jansen)
* Moderately potent—Betnovate N (betamethasone and neomycin) (Glaxo); Synalar N (neomycin; Zeneca)
  —Trimovate cream (clobetasone butyrate, nystatin and oxytetracycline; Glaxo)
  —Fucibet (betamethasone, fucidic acid; Leo)
* Very potent   —Dermovate-NN (clobetasone, with neomycin and nystatin; Glaxo).

Antiseptics and cleaning lotions

Simple antiseptics are very useful for cleaning infected, weeping lesions and leg ulcers.

Potassium permanganate can be used by dropping four or five crystals in a litre of water or in an 0·1% solution that is diluted to 0·01% for use as a soak. It will stain the skin temporarily and plastic containers permanently.

Silver nitrate 0·25% is a simple, safe antiseptic solution that, applied as a wet compress, is useful for cleaning ulcers.

Flamazine (Smith and Nephew) is silver sulphadiazine cream, used for leg ulcers, pressure sores, and burns.

Hydrogen peroxide (6%) helps remove slough but tends to be painful. Hioxyl (Quinoderm) is a proprietary cream for desloughing.

Iodine (2.5%) is an old fashioned effective preparation as a tincture in alcohol and Betadine (Napp) is a proprietary equivalent.

Shampoos containing septrimide-caenal, quinoderm, and povidone iodine (Betadine Seton), selinium sulphide (Selsun Abbot) or ketoconazole (Nizoral, Jansenn) for tinea versicolor and seborrhoeic dermatitis.

There are numerous other antiseptic, cleansing, and desloughing agents such as cetrimide, chlorhexidine, benzalkonium chloride, benzoic acid, and enzyme preparations such as Varidase (Lederle), a streptokinase and streptodornase preparation.

Special situations

Keratolytics, for hyperkeratoses—salicylic acid 2–4% in aqueous cream—salicylic acid with betamethasone ointment (Diprosalic ointment, Schering-Plough).

Anti-pruritics, for persistent itching—menthol (0·5%) or phenol 1% in aqueous cream—calamine lotion.

Antiperspirants, aluminium chloride for hyperhydrosis, aluminium chloride 20% (Driclor, Stiefel or anhydrol, Dermal Laboratories).

Depigmenting agents—2% hydroquinone cream available without prescription as "fade-out".

Preparations for the mouth—Adcortyl in Orabase (Squibb) or Corlan pellets (Evans). Both these preparations contain corticosteroids. Daktarin (Jansen) or Fungilin lozenges (Squibb), Nystan (nystatin suspension, Squibb). All these preparations are antifungal.

Preparations for treating acne and varicose ulcers are described in the appropriate sections.

Further reading

Arndt KA. *Manual of dermatological therapeutics.* 5th ed. New York: Little, 1995.
Barker DJ, Millard LG. *Essentials of skin disease management.* Oxford: Blackwell Scientific, 1979.
Lamberg SI. *Dermatology in primary care: a problem oriented guide.* Philadelphia: Saunders, 1986.
Stone LA, Lindfield EM, Robertson SJ. *A colour atlas of nursing procedures in skin disorders.* London: Wolfe, 1989.

Index

Page numbers printed in **bold** type refer to illustrations; those in *italic* to boxed material

Index

Index

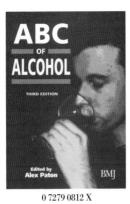
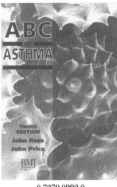
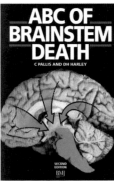
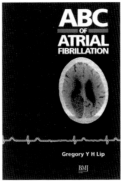
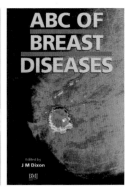
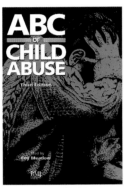
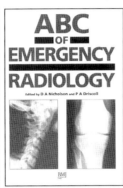
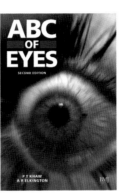
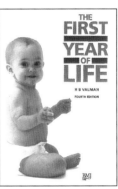
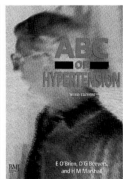
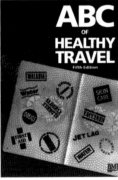
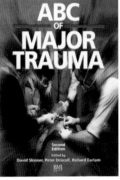
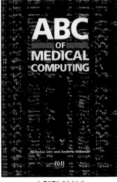
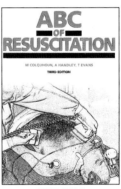
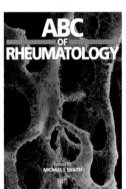
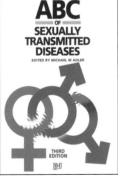
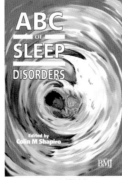
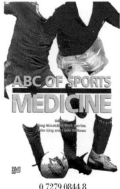
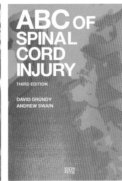
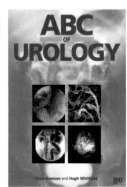
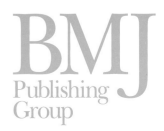